Advances in Diagnosis and Treatment of Peritoneum Cancer

Advances in Diagnosis and Treatment of Peritoneum Cancer

Guest Editors

Manuel Diez-Alonso

Alberto Gutierrez-Calvo

MDPI

Basel • Beijing • Wuhan • Barcelona • Belgrade • Novi Sad • Cluj • Manchester

Guest Editors
Manuel Diez-Alonso
Department of General
Surgery
Príncipe de Asturias
University Hospital
Alcalá de Henares
Spain

Alberto Gutierrez-Calvo
Department of General
Surgery
Príncipe de Asturias
University Hospital
Alcalá de Henares
Spain

Editorial Office
MDPI AG
Grosspeteranlage 5
4052 Basel, Switzerland

This is a reprint of the Special Issue, published open access by the journal *Journal of Clinical Medicine* (ISSN 2077-0383), freely accessible at: https://www.mdpi.com/journal/jcm/special_issues/8H581974RF.

For citation purposes, cite each article independently as indicated on the article page online and as indicated below:

Lastname, A.A.; Lastname, B.B. Article Title. *Journal Name* **Year**, *Volume Number*, Page Range.

ISBN 978-3-7258-4603-0 (Hbk)
ISBN 978-3-7258-4604-7 (PDF)
https://doi.org/10.3390/books978-3-7258-4604-7

Contents

Journal of
Clinical Medicine

Editorial

Peritoneal Metastases: Evolution from a Dark Horizon to an Encouraging Present and a Promising Future

Manuel Diez-Alonso [1,*], Alberto San-Juan [2], Miguel Angel Ortega [3] and Alberto Gutiérrez-Calvo [1]

1 General Surgery Service, University Hospital Príncipe de Asturias, 28820 Alcalá de Henares, Spain; alberto.gutierrez@salud.madrid.org
2 Medical Oncology Service, University Hospital Príncipe de Asturias, 28820 Alcalá de Henares, Spain; albsanjuan_2@hotmail.com
3 Department of Medicine and Medical Specialities, Faculty of Medicine and Health Sciences, University of Alcalá de Henares, 28880 Alcala de Henares, Spain; miguel.angel.ortega92@gmail.com
* Correspondence: manuelmariano.diez@salud.madrid.org

Peritoneal metastasis (PM) is the primary pattern of metastasis for primary tumours of the appendix, ovary, and peritoneal mesothelioma. There is a modest risk of PM in patients with colorectal or gastric cancer; however, it is much less common in patients with other tumours, such as soft tissue sarcoma, breast cancer, melanoma, and lung cancer [1]. Traditionally, the presence of PM has been considered an incurable situation; after their diagnosis, patients were informed that their prognosis was only a few months and that there was no effective treatment. The survival of patients with PM is poorer than that of patients with metastases in other sites, such as the liver or lungs. Additionally, it is known that the survival of patients with metastasis decreases if the peritoneum is affected. In fact, the eighth actualisation of the American Joint Committee on Cancer's (AJCC) TNM classification system for Colorectal Cancer, published in 2016, established a new M1 subclass named M1c in order to include patients with PM due to their poor prognosis of survival. However, during recent years, a number of significant therapeutic contributions have opened an expectancy of a promising future so that this condition may no longer be considered a death sentence [1–3]. Several factors have contributed to this change. Our knowledge about the biology of peritoneal disease, its clinical behaviour, and the prognostic factors for survival has progressed, and we know that it is not a uniform disease. the introduction of modern chemotherapeutic drugs and biologically targeted agents, with superior cytotoxic efficacy and less toxic effects, have also changed the treatment [1–5]. In addition, cytoreductive surgery (CRS), either accompanied or unaccompanied by hyperthermic intraperitoneal chemotherapy (HIPEC), has been introduced for the treatment of patients with PM with promising results and a great degree of acceptance. Thus, PM can no longer be considered as a process with an inevitable lethal end.

In approximately 25% of cases, PM appears as the sole presentation site of metastatic disease. Most patients diagnosed with PM undergo systemic treatment with chemotherapy; however, CRS with or without HIPEC is a reasonable option in patients with low-risk comorbidities and a low-to-moderate extent of peritoneal dissemination [6]. However, CRS/HIPEC possesses high morbidity and mortality rates, and the careful selection of candidates is mandatory.

According to Lambert in a recent review, the first clinical communication of the application of CRS/HIPEC was made by Spratt in 1980 [1]. This author described the technique used for the treatment of a case of PM originating from an appendiceal mucinous neoplasm and described the concept of "peritoneal surface malignancy" as well as the basis for the treatment of PM as a regional disease. EVOCAPE [7] was the first clinical study indicating that some patients with PM could obtain benefit if they are treated with CRS/HIPEC. In that study, when CRS/HIPEC plus multimodal therapy (surgery and best systemic chemotherapy) was used for colorectal, appendiceal, or ovarian cancers, the median survival improved; conversely, similar results could not be reproduced for primary tumours of the pancreas, hepatobiliary organs, and other foregut organs. This trial effectively promoted a new and contemporary surgical approach for patients with resectable PM. However, the technique spread and became generalised thanks to the works and publications of Sugarbaker [6].

CRS/HIPEC has been associated with controversy for years, and its implementation has not been easy. The small number of randomised clinical trials, the difficulty and degree of skill required by the surgical technique, the morbidity associated with the procedure, the lack of homogeneity in its application (open vs. closed HIPEC; HIPEC vs. PIPAC; the selection of perfused chemotherapy), and the lack of knowledge of the contribution of each of the two components (cytoreduction vs. chemotherapy) have contributed to persistent doubts about its efficacy. However, CRS/HIPEC is currently fully accepted, and it is implemented in today's daily clinical practice throughout the world. Given the limited amount of solid evidence derived from scientifically proven data, the rationale that justifies the use of CRS/HIPEC is based, for the most part, on retrospective and uncontrolled studies. Currently, CRS/HIPEC is the first option of treatment in patients with low-grade mucinous tumours of the appendix, in advanced ovarian tumours, and in patients with colorectal cancer or peritoneal mesothelioma with a low tumour burden (PCI < 20).

The first randomised trial designed to analyse the role of CRS in patients with PM from Colorectal Cancer was conducted in the Netherlands between 1990 and 1998 [8]. It compared 5 FU/palliative surgery versus 5 FU/CRS/HIPEC plus mitomycin C for 90 min at 40.5 °C. Although the size of the analysed sample was very small (105 patients), the obtained results indicated that survival was better in the CRS/HIPEC arm (22.4 months versus 12.6 months) ($p = 0.032$). A French group proposed and reported good results with the use of HIPEC with a perfusion of oxaliplatin for 30 min [9]. This regimen was recently tested in the PRODIGE 7 trial [10], in which the median overall survival was similar in the CRS/HIPEC group (41·7 months) and in the CRS-on ly group (41·2 months). However, this study reported the longest survival in patients with CRC-PM survival at 42 months, demonstrating the benefit of combining the best systemic therapy with CRS. The currently ongoing CAIRO6 trial [11] is exploring the therapeutic benefit of combining systemic perioperative chemotherapy with CRS/HIPEC.

Two lines of research have explored the efficacy of using CRS/HIPEC for the treatment of PM in an initial or subclinical phase. HIPECT4 [12] explored the use of CRS/HIPEC for 60 min with mitomycin C in a prophylactic setting in patients staged as cT4/N0-2/M0 at diagnosis. The conclusions and relevance obtained were that the addition of HIPEC to CRS improved the 3-year locoregional control rate compared with surgery alone. COLOPEC2 [13] analysed the use of an exploratory laparoscopy during the follow -up in pT4 colon cancer patients for the early detection of peritoneal metastases, at 1 month and at 18 months, compared with computed tomographic imaging. This study was designed to detect occult peritoneal disease that was not identified in the COLOPEC [14] and PROPHYOCHIP trials [15].

The OVHIPEC randomised trial evaluated the efficacy of HIPEC in chemotherapy-naive cases of advanced ovarian cancer [16]. Patients received three cycles of neoadjuvant carboplatin/paclitaxel and were randomised to receive either CRS alone or CRS/HIPEC with a perfusion of cisplatin during 90 min of HIPEC, followed by adjuvant chemotherapy. Better progression-free survival and overall survival were observed in the CRS/HIPEC arm.

Not only have surgical procedures evolved [17], but chemotherapy and systemic agents have also contributed to improve the prognoses of PM patients. There are many different novel treatments that have been introduced in recent years and have been approved for the metastases of different tumours, such as antiangiogenic agents, monoclonal antibodies, and biologic or immune modulator drugs or targeted treatments, that have clearly contributed to better response rates, progression-free survival, and overall survival.

Bevacizumab and Aflibercept are two antibodies that act against the Vascular Endothelial Growth Factor that, when combined with chemotherapy, prolong overall survival beyond 24 months in colorectal cancer patients, independent of their RAS statuses. Cetuximab and Panitumumab are monoclonal antibodies that act against the Epidermal Growth Factor Receptor on the cell membrane in tumours with a non-mutated KRAS gene, which blocks the growth of tumour cells. It is known that these types of drugs reduce the progression of various types of tumours, such as colorectal cancer. In addition, the drugs regorafenib and TAS-112 have emerged as third-line or beyond treatments for colorectal tumours and provide improved overall survival.

The incidence of tumours that express microsatellite instability is very low, but this small group of patients could be treated with immunotherapy, with high response rates, survival, and quality of life, without many of the potential severe adverse effects that are associated with chemotherapy treatment. The TOGA trial [18] revealed that HER-2-positive advanced gastric tumours could benefit from the addition of trastuzumab to 5-FU/platinum-based agents. The median overall survival of patients receiving trastuzumab plus chemotherapy was higher than that observed in patients treated with chemotherapy alone (13.8 vs. 11.1 months). ATTRACTION-4 [19] was a randomised, multicentre, double-blind trial that explored the combination of nivolumab with oxaliplatin-based chemotherapy, and it observed significantly improved progression-free survival.

In the treatment of advanced ovarian cancer, there has been critical innovation with the introduction of PARP inhibitors (olaparib, niraparib, and veliparib) as maintenance therapy for stage III/IV after CRS. PARP is an enzyme involved in the repair of damaged DNA that has been identified as a target in cancers that have BRCA1/BRCA2 mutations and/or recombination repair deficiency [20,21].

These different options in the treatment of PM have become an encouraging challenge for medical oncologists; they should choose the best treatment strategy early in the course of the disease and consider the preferred regimens for each stage of the disease to provide patients with the longest survival and best quality of life possible. The clinical management of PM still entails many difficulties, and depending on the type of primary tumour, different therapeutic approaches are available.

There has been a revolution in the treatment of patients with PM as new and different avenues of research have been opened and progress has been made. What could be the roles of laparoscopy and robotic surgery in the future? How can the new modalities of magnetic resonance imaging contribute to the earlier detection and staging of PM? Future developments in molecular profiling methods will allow for the identification of precise molecular changes that are responsible for PM. Advances in immunotherapy, where immune checkpoint inhibitors and other immunotherapeutic strategies are now being studied, have made it a promising option. Drug delivery systems based on nanotechnology have the ability to deliver chemotherapeutic drugs to tumour cells within the peritoneal cavity in a targeted and regulated manner. This strategy could reduce systemic toxicity while increasing the effectiveness of chemotherapy. Another promising strategy to identify the response to therapy and for the early detection of recurrence is the identification of circulating tumour cells. In the future, we will know if it could be a useful tool to improve survival.

Conflicts of Interest: The authors declare no conflict of interest.

References

1. Lambert, L.A. Looking Up: Recent Advances in Understanding and treating Peritoneal Carcinomatosis. *CA Cancer J. Clin.* **2015**, *65*, 283–298. [CrossRef] [PubMed]
2. Baaten, I.C.P.A.; West, N.P.; Quyn, A.J.; Seymour, M.T.; Seligmann, J.F. Colorectal cancer peritoneal metastases: Biology, treatment and next steps. *Eur. J. Surg. Oncol.* **2020**, *46*, 675–683. [CrossRef] [PubMed]
3. Sánchez-Hidalgo, J.M.; Rodríguez-Ortiz, L.; Arjona-Sánchez, Á.; Rufián-Peña, S.; Casado-Adam, Á.; Cosano-Álvarez, A.; Briceño-Delgado, J. Colorectal peritoneal metastases: Optimal management review. *World J. Gastroenterol.* **2019**, *25*, 3484–3502. [CrossRef] [PubMed]

4. Van Cutsem, E.; Cervantes, A.; Adam, R.; Sobrero, A.; Van Krieken, J.H.; Aderka, D.; Aguilar, E.A.; Bardelli, A.; Benson, A.; Bodoky, G.; et al. ESMO consensus guidelines for the management of patients with metastatic colorectal cancer. *Ann. Oncol.* **2016**, *27*, 1386–1422. [CrossRef] [PubMed]
5. Sanoff, H.K.; Sargent, D.J.; Campbell, M.E.; Morton, R.F.; Fuchs, C.S.; Ramanathan, R.K.; Williamson, S.K.; Findlay, B.P.; Pitot, H.C.; Goldberg, R.M. Five-year data and prognostic factor Analysis of oxaliplatin and irinotecan combinations for advanced colorectal cancer: N9741. *J. Clin. Oncol.* **2008**, *26*, 5721–5727. [CrossRef] [PubMed]
6. Sugarbaker, P.H.; Jablonski, K.A. Prognostic features of 51 colorectal and 130 appendiceal cáncer patients with peritoneal carcinomatosis treated by cytoreductive surgery and intraperitoneal chemotherapy. *Ann. Surg.* **1995**, *221*, 124–132. [CrossRef]
7. Sadeghi, B.; Arvieux, C.; Glehen, O.; Beaujard, A.D.; Rivoire, M.; Baulieux, J.; Fontaumard, E.; Brachet, A.; Caillot, J.L.; Faure, J.L.; et al. Peritoneal carcinomatosis from nongynecologic malignancies: Results of the EVOCAPE 1 multicentric prospective study. *Cancer* **2000**, *88*, 358–363. [CrossRef]
8. Verwaal, V.J.; van Ruth, S.; de Bree, E.; van Slloothen, G.W.; van Tinteren, H.; Boot, H.; Zoetmulder, F.A. Randomized trial of cytoreduction and hyperthermic intraperitoneal chemotherapy and palliative surgery in patients with peritoneal carcinomatosis of colorrectal cáncer. *J. Clin. Oncol.* **2003**, *21*, 3737–3743. [CrossRef]
9. Quenet, F.; Goeze, D.; Mehta, S.S.; Roca, L.; Dumont, F.; Hessissen, M.; Saint-Aubert, B.; Elias, D. Results of two bi-institutional prospective studies using intraperitoneal oxaliplatin with or without irinotecan during HIPEC after cytoreductive surgery for colorectal carcinomatosis. *Ann. Surg.* **2011**, *254*, 294–301. [CrossRef]
10. Quenet, F.; Elias, D.; Roca, L.; Goere, D.; Ghouti, L.; Pocard, M.; Facy, M.; Arvieux, C.; Lorimier, G.; Pezet, D.; et al. Cytoreductive surgery plus hyperthermic intraperitoneal chemotherapy versus cytoreductive surgery alone for colorectal peritoneal metastases (PRODIGE 7): A multicentre, randomised, open-label, phase 3 trial. *Lancet Oncol.* **2011**, *22*, 256–266. [CrossRef]
11. Rovers, K.P.; Bakkers, C.; Nienhuijs, S.W.; Burger, J.W.A.; Creemers, G.M.; Thijs, A.M.J.; Brandt-Kerkhof, A.R.M.; Madsen, E.V.E.; van Meerten, E.; Tuynman, J.B.; et al. Perioperative systemic therapy and cytoreductive surgery with HIPEC versus upfront cytoreductive surgery with HIPEC alone for isolated resectable colorectal peritoneal metastases: Protocol of a multicentre, open-label, parallel-group, phase II-II, randomised, superiority study (CAIRO6). *JAMA Surg.* **2021**, *156*, 710–720.
12. Arjona-Sánchez, A.; Espinosa-Redondo, E.; Gutiérrez-Calvo, A.; Segura-Sampedro, J.; Pérez-Viejo, S.; Martín, V.C.; Sánchez García, S.; García-Fadrique, A.; Prieto-Nieto, I.; Barrios-Sanchez, P.; et al. Efficacy and Safety of Intraoperative Hyperthermic Intraperitoneal Chemotherapy for Locally Advanced Colon Cancer A Phase 3 Randomized Clinical Trial. *JAMA Surg.* **2023**, *158*, 683–691. [CrossRef]
13. Bastiaenen, V.P.; Klaver, C.E.L.; Kok, N.F.M.; de Wilt, J.H.W.; de Hingh, I.H.J.T.; Aalbers, A.G.J.; Boerma, D.; Bremers, A.J.A.; Burger, J.W.A.; van Duyn, E.B.; et al. Second and third look laparoscopy in pT4 colon cancer patients for early detection of peritoneal metastases; the COLOPEC2 randomized multicentre trial. *BMC Cancer* **2019**, *19*, 254. [CrossRef]
14. Klaver, C.E.L.; Wisselink, D.D.; Punt, C.J.A.; Snaebjornsson, P.; Crezee, J.; Aalbers, A.G.J.; Brandt, A.; Bremers, A.J.A.; Burger, J.W.A.; Fabry, H.F.J.; et al. Adjuvant hyperthermic intraperitoneal chemotherapy in patients with locally advanced colon cancer (COLOPEC): A multicentre, open-label, randomised trial. *Lancet Gastroenterol. Hepatol.* **2019**, *4*, 716–770. [CrossRef] [PubMed]
15. Goéré, D.; Glehen, O.; Quenet, F.; Guilloit, J.M.; Bereder, J.M.; Lorimier, G.; Thibaudeau, E.; Ghouti, L.; Pinto, A.; Tuech, J.J.; et al. Second-look surgery plus hyperthermic intraperitoneal chemotherapy versus surveillance in patients at high risk of developing colorrectal peritoneal metastases (PROPHYLOCHIP-PRODIGE 15): A randomised, phase 3 study. *Lancet Oncol.* **2020**, *21*, 1147–1154. [CrossRef] [PubMed]
16. van Driel, W.J.; Koole, S.N.; Sikorska, K.; Schagen van Leeuwen, J.H.; Schreuder, H.W.R.; Hermans, R.H.M.; de Hingh, I.H.J.T.; van der Velden, J.; Arts, H.J.; Massuger, L.F.A.G.; et al. Hyperthermic intraperitoneal chemotherapy in ovarian cancer. *N. Engl. J. Med.* **2018**, *378*, 230–240. [CrossRef] [PubMed]
17. Sugarbaker, P.H. Peritonectomy procedures. *Ann. Surg.* **1995**, *221*, 29–42. [CrossRef] [PubMed]
18. Van Cutsem, E.; Bang, Y.J.; Feng-yi, F.; Xu, J.M.; Lee, K.W.; Jiao, S.C.; Chong, J.L.; Lopez-Sanchez, R.; Price, T.; Gladkov, O.; et al. HER2 screening data from ToGA: Targeting HER2 in gastric and gastroesophageal junction cancer. HER2 screening data from TOGA: Targeting HER2 in gastric and gastroesophageal junction cancer. *Gastric Cancer* **2015**, *18*, 476–484. [CrossRef] [PubMed]
19. Kang, Y.K.; Chen, L.T.; Ryu, M.H.; Oh, D.Y.; Oh, S.C.; Chung, H.C.; Lee, K.W.; Omori, T.; Shitara, K.; Sakuramoto, S.; et al. Nivolumab plus chemotherapy versus placebo plus chemotherapy in patients with HER2-negative, untreated, unresectable advanced or recurrent gastric or gastro-oesophageal junction cancer (ATTRACTION-4): A randomised, multicentre, double-blind, placebo-controlled, phase 3 trial. *Lancet Oncol.* **2022**, *23*, 234–247. [PubMed]
20. Mirza, M.R.; Coleman, R.L.; González-Martín, A.; Moore, K.N.; Colombo, N.; Ray-Coquard, I.; Pignata, S. The forefront of ovarian cancer therapy: Update on PARP inhibitors. *Ann. Oncol.* **2020**, *31*, 1148–1159. [CrossRef]
21. Lorusso, D.; Guy, H.; Samyshkin, Y.; Hawkes, C.; Estenson, K.; Coleman, R.L. Feasibility Study of a Network Meta-Analysis and Unanchored Population-Adjusted Indirect Treatment Comparison of Niraparib, Olaparib, and Bevacizumab as Maintenance Therapies in Patients with Newly Diagnosed Advanced Ovarian Cancer. *Cancers* **2022**, *14*, 1285. [CrossRef] [PubMed]

Journal of
Clinical Medicine

MDPI

Article

Initial Experience of Cytoreductive Surgery (CRS) and Hyperthermic Intraperitoneal Chemotherapy (HIPEC) in Baltic Country Center

Rokas Račkauskas *, Augustinas Baušys, Jonas Jurgaitis, Marius Paškonis and Kęstutis Strupas

Clinic of Gastroenterology, Nephrourology, and Surgery, Institute of Clinical Medicine, Faculty of Medicine, Vilnius University, Ciurlionio Str. 21, 03101 Vilnius, Lithuania
* Correspondence: rokas.rackauskas@santa.lt; Tel.: +370-60190691

Abstract: Background: Peritoneal surface malignancies (PSMs) are a heterogenous group of primary and metastatic cancers affecting the peritoneum. They are associated with poor long-term outcomes. Many centers around the world adopt cytoreductive surgery (CRS) and hyperthermic intraperitoneal chemotherapy (HIPEC) in routine clinical practice for these otherwise condemned patients despite a lack of high-level evidence from randomized control trials. This study aimed to investigate and present our 10-year experience with this controversial method, CRS and HIPEC, for PSM in a single tertiary center in a Baltic country. **Methods:** Patients who underwent CRS and HIPEC at Vilnius University Hospital Santaros Klinikos between 2011 and 2021 were included in this retrospective study. Overall survival was the primary study outcome. Secondary outcomes included postoperative morbidity and mortality, and local or systemic recurrence rates. **Results:** Sixty-nine patients who underwent CRS and HIPEC were included in the study. Most patients underwent treatment for peritoneal metastases from colorectal, ovarian, and appendiceal cancers. Six (8.7%) patients received CRS and HIPEC for primary peritoneal neoplasm—pseudomyxoma peritonei. The mean peritoneal carcinomatosis index score was 12 ± 7. Complete cytoreduction was achieved in 62 (89.9%) patients. The mean OS was 39 ± 29 months. The mean survival of patients with PSMs of different origin was as follows: 39 ± 25 (95% CI: 28–50) months for colorectal cancer, 44 ± 31 (95% CI: 30–58) months for ovarian cancer, 32 ± 21 (95% CI: 21–43) months for appendiceal cancer, 422 ± 1 (95% CI: 12–97) months for pseudomyxoma peritonei, and 7 months for gastric cancer. **Conclusions:** The current study demonstrated the results of the CRS and HIPEC program in a single Baltic country tertiary center. Patients who underwent CRS and HIPEC for PSMs achieved moderate survival rates with acceptable postoperative morbidity and mortality risk.

Keywords: peritoneal surface malignancies; cytoreductive surgery; hyperthermic intraperitoneal chemotherapy; Peritoneal mesothelioma; colorectal peritoneal metastases; peritoneal carcinomatosis; peritoneum cancer

1. Background

Peritoneal mesothelioma, pseudomyxoma peritonei, and peritoneal metastases of various cancers are among the main tumors that make up the heterogeneous group of peritoneal surface malignancies (PSMs). The most typical sources of metastasis are colorectal, stomach, and ovarian malignancies [1]. Irrespective of the origin, PSMs are associated with poor long-term outcomes. Historically, the main treatment options for PSM patients were palliative systemic chemotherapy or palliative care [2,3]. However, in recent decades, the notion of futile PSM treatment has evolved. The oncological community has grown interested in a more aggressive and potentially curative treatment approach using cytoreductive surgery (CRS) and hyperthermic intraperitoneal chemotherapy (HIPEC) [4]. Many centers around the world adopt CRS and HIPEC in routine clinical practice for these otherwise condemned patients despite a lack of high-level evidence from randomized control trials

(RCTs). Accumulating evidence from observational studies promoted the spread of CRS and HIPEC for PSMs, and now, the treatment is considered the standard of care for primary peritoneal malignancies despite the absence of level 1 evidence due to lack of an effective alternative treatment [5]. However, certain recent high-quality RCTs, such as PRODIGE7, COLOPEC, CYTO-CHIP, and PROFILOCHIP presented conflicting data and questioned whether HIPEC regimens currently in use are helpful for peritoneal metastases [6–9]. Thus, this study aimed to investigate and present our 10-year experience with this controversial method, CRS and HIPEC, for PSMs in a single tertiary center in a Baltic country.

2. Materials and Methods

2.1. Ethics

Ethical approval from Vilnius regional biomedical research ethics committee (No. 2020/11-1279-761) was obtained before the start of the study. The waiver for informed consent was given by the authority. The study was conducted according to the Declaration of Helsinki.

2.2. Patients and Data Collection

All consecutive patients who underwent CRS and HIPEC at Vilnius University Hospital Santaros Klinikos between 2011 and 2021 were included in this retrospective study. Every patient with a PSM was discussed at multidisciplinary team meetings and decision to perform CRS and HIPEC for PSMs was individualized depending on patients' general condition (ECOG 0-1), etiology, and the dissemination of the disease. Data on patient characteristics were extracted from the prospectively collected institutional electronic database. They included clinicopathologic characteristics (age; gender; history of previous cancer treatment; origin, number, and size of metastatic lesions; and peritoneal carcinomatosis index (PCI) score) and treatment-related characteristics (length of surgery; blood loss; HIPEC regime; postoperative complications as per Clavien–Dindo classification).

2.3. Study Outcomes

The primary outcome of the study was overall survival (OS) in patients with peritoneal carcinomatosis treated with CRS and HIPEC. OS was defined as the time from surgical intervention to death. The secondary outcomes included postoperative morbidity, mortality, and local or systemic recurrence. Data on survival and date of death were collected from the Lithuanian National Cancer Registry.

2.4. CRS and HIPEC Regimens

All procedures were performed under general anesthesia. At first, laparotomy was performed, and the extent of CRS and organ resections depended on the dissemination of the disease. After CRS, HIPEC was performed. Different protocols were used for PSMs of different origin:

1. For ovarian and gastric cancer, the HIPEC protocol consisted of Cisplatin at 75 mg/m^2 with 4 L of 0.9% saline at 42 °C for 60 min;
2. For colorectal cancer, the HIPEC protocol consisted of Oxaliplatin at 460/m^2 with 4 L of 5% glucose at 42 °C for 45 min until 2017; later, it was changed to Mytomicin C at 30 mg + 10 mg, with 5 L of 1.5% dextrose at 42 °C for 90 min;
3. For primary PSMs (pseudomyxoma peritonei, appendiceal cancer), the HIPEC protocol consisted of Mytomicin C 30 mg + 10 mg, with 5-L 1.5% dextrose at 42 °C for 90 min.

After surgery, all patients were moved to the intensive care unit for further treatment. Typically, if patients vital functions were stable, they were moved to further treatment in a surgical ward on postoperative day 1 or 2.

2.5. Statistical Analysis

All statistical analyses were conducted using the statistical program SPSS 24.0 (SPSS, Chicago, IL, USA). Continuous variables are presented as means with standard deviation and an interquartile range. Categorical variables are shown as proportions. Continuous variables were compared using a Mann–Whitney U-test and categorical variables with Pearson's chi-square or Fisher's exact test, as appropriate. Overall survival rates were using the Kaplan–Meier method and compared with the log-rank test. Statistical significance was considered when a p-value < 0.05 was achieved.

3. Results

3.1. Baseline Characteristics

In total, 69 patients who underwent CRS and HIPEC were included in the study. The baseline characteristics of patients are shown in Table 1. All patients (100%) had an ASA score of 2 or 3. Most patients underwent treatment for peritoneal metastases from colorectal, ovarian, and appendiceal cancers. Six (8.7%) patients received CRS and HIPEC for primary peritoneal neoplasm—pseudomyxoma peritonei. The mean peritoneal carcinomatosis index (PCI) score at the time of surgery was 12 ± 7. Complete cytoreduction was achieved in 62 (89.9%) patients. After CRS and HIPEC, all patients (100%) received systemic therapy (chemotherapy/biological therapy) prior and after the procedure

Table 1. Baseline clinicopathologic characteristics of patients who underwent cytoreductive surgery and hyperthermic intraperitoneal chemotherapy for peritoneal surface malignancies.

Characteristics of HIPEC Patients		
Sex	Female (n; %)	56 (81.2%)
	Male (n; %)	13 (18.8%)
Mean age ± SD (Q1; Q3), years		57.2 ± 10.89 (49; 67)
Mean hospitalization ± SD (Q1; Q3), days		20.19 ± 14.69 (12; 23.5)
Peritoneal histology (n; %): Colorectal Ovarian Appendiceal: - LAMN - HAMN Pseudomyxoma peritonei Gastric		 22 (31.9%) 23 (33.3%) 17 (24.6%) 13 (18.8%) 4 (5.8%) 6 (8.7%) 1 (1.4%)
Mean PCI score ± SD (Q1; Q3)		12.2 ± 7.6 (6.25; 15.75)
Mean operation time ± SD (Q1; Q3), min		447.5 ± 152.7 (310; 540)
Mean blood loss ± SD (Q1; Q3), mL		350.7 ± 284.3 (200.0; 500.0)
Cytoreduction completeness: - CC0 (n; %) - CC1 (n; %) - CC2 (n; %)		 - 62 (89.9%) - 6 (8.7%) - 1 (1.4%)
Complications C–D: - No complications - <3 - 3a - 3b - 5		 36 (52.2%) 21 (30.4%) 5 (7.2%) 6 (8.7%) 1 (1.4%)

3.2. Postoperative Morbidity

Postoperative complications occurred in 33 (47.8%) patients, including 11 patients (15.9%) who suffered severe complications (≥Clavien–Dindo 3). The postoperative mortality rate was 1.4% (one patient). A detailed list of complications and their severity according to the Clavien–Dindo classification is shown in Table 2.

Table 2. Postoperative complications after cytoreductive surgery and hyperthermic intraperitoneal chemotherapy for peritoneal surface malignancies.

Complication	Number of Patients	C–D
Atrial fibrillation	2	1
Wound infection	6	2
Urinary tract infection	3	2
Renal insufficiency	3	1
Pancytopenia	2	2
Hydrothorax	5	2
Pneumonia	3	2
Intraabdominal abscess	4	3a
Intraabdominal bleeding	1	3b
Pancreatic fistula	2	3a
Ileus	3	1
Anastomotic leakage	5	3b
Compartment syndrome	1	3b
Postoperative myocardial infarction	1	5

3.3. Long-Term Outcomes

The mean OS of patients treated with CRS and HIPEC was 39 ± 29 months; however, it greatly depended on the etiology of the disease. The mean survival of patients with PSMs of different origin was as follows: 39 ± 25 (95% CI: 28–50) months for colorectal cancer, 44 ± 31 (95% CI: 30–58) months for ovarian cancer, 32 ± 21 (95% CI: 21–43) months for appendiceal cancer, 42 ± 21 (95% CI: 12–97) months for pseudomyxoma peritonei, and 7 months for gastric cancer. However, these differences failed for significance (Figure 1). The mean time for recurrence was 15 ± 12 months, with no differences among PSMs of different origin (data not shown).

3.4. CRS and HIPEC Development in the Study Center

Since the implementation of CRS and HIPEC into clinical practice at our center, there have been ongoing worldwide debates about the effectiveness and benefits of this treatment modality. However, through the study period, with accumulating high-level evidence questioning the effectiveness of CRS and HIPEC in many cancers, the number of procedures tended to drop at our center (Figure 2). Currently, CRS and HIPEC are performed at our center only for primary peritoneal malignancy and appendiceal LAMN and HAMN tumors.

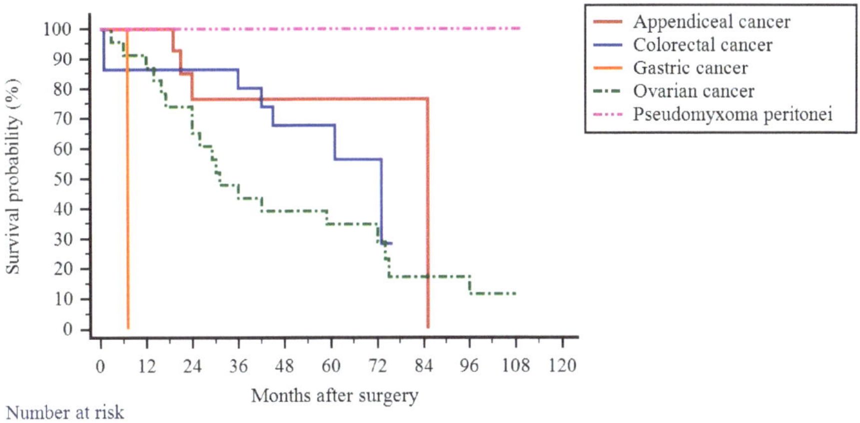

Number at risk

Group	0	12	24	36	48	60	72	84	96	108	120
Appendiceal cancer	17	15	9	5	3	2	1	1	0	0	0
Colorectal cancer	22	17	15	13	10	6	2	0	0	0	0
Gastric cancer	1	0	0	0	0	0	0	0	0	0	0
Ovarian cancer	23	20	15	10	9	8	5	3	2	0	0
Pseudomyxoma peritonei	6	4	2	2	2	2	2	2	2	1	0

Figure 1. Overall survival of patients who underwent cytoreductive surgery and hyperthermic intraperitoneal chemotherapy for peritoneal surface malignancies.

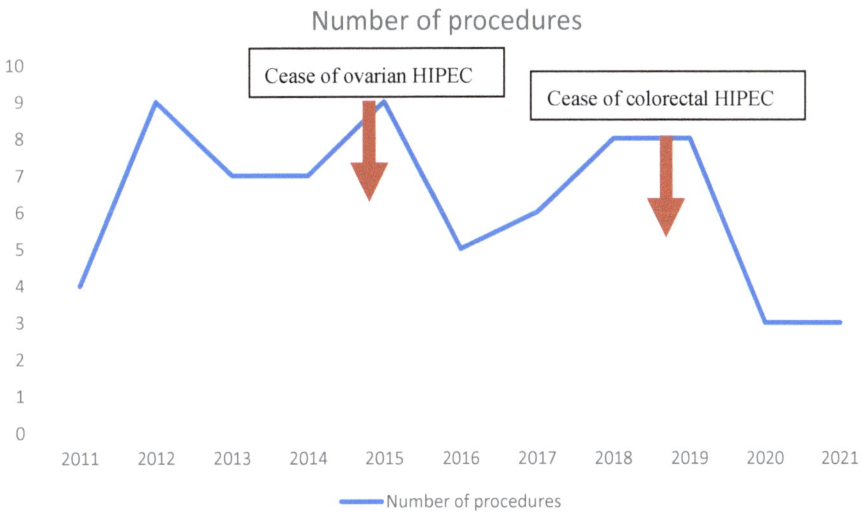

Figure 2. The annual number of cytoreductive surgery and hyperthermic intraperitoneal chemotherapy procedures throughout the study period.

4. Discussion

The present study demonstrated the results of CRS and HIPEC for PSMs at a single tertiary center in a Baltic country. The postoperative outcomes achieved in our study in terms of postoperative morbidity and long-term outcomes are comparable to international standards. The present study showed that CRS and HIPEC are safe and feasible with a low mortality rate in medium- or low-volume centers in small-population countries. However, current standard indications for CRS and HIPEC are narrow; thus, clinical trials may be an option to offer this treatment to patients and maintain sufficient center volume.

Since the introduction of CRS and HIPEC for PSMs, it has been postulated to increase the survival of patients with advanced peritoneal surface disease [10,11]. However, recent RCTs showed controversial results, and the rationale for HIPEC in some types of cancer became questionable. The third most prevalent disease in the world is colorectal cancer, and up to 15% of patients have peritoneal metastases [12]. The present study showed that CRS and HIPEC in such patients can achieve a mean survival of 39 months. Such results seem promising, similar to initial reports that showed that CRS and HIPEC offer survival benefits over systemic chemotherapy [13]. However, a recent PRODIGE-7 study showed that HIPEC did not improve survival in colorectal cancer patients who achieved CC0 resection compared with CRS alone but increased morbidity 60 days after surgery. Thus, our satisfactory results achieved using CRS and HIPEC do not encourage the further adoption of the method for colorectal cancer patients [6,14].

Another entity that may be considered for CRS and HIPEC is ovarian cancer. In our study, these patients achieved a mean survival of 44 months. Globally, there are still ongoing debates regarding HIPEC's role after CRS for primary and recurrent ovarian cancer [15,16]. Some studies showed that patients with stage III epithelial ovarian cancer may benefit from HIPEC after CRS in terms of increased OS and recurrence-free survival [17]. However, the lack of robust evidence resulted in a decreased number of these procedures for ovarian cancer in our center [18].

Primary peritoneal malignancies, such as pseudomyxoma peritonei or malignant mesothelioma, and mucinous appendiceal tumors are among those where CRS with HIPEC is the standard treatment option [19]. Several studies comparing CRS with HIPEC to surgery and debulking alone failed to show HIPEC benefits for long-term outcomes [20,21], but the lack of an effective alternative treatment still precludes abandoning HIPEC for these patients. Thus, the recent clinical practice guidelines recommend that patients with these rare malignancies should be referred to a specialized center for a personalized treatment approach [22]. In our center's experience, CRS and HIPEC are feasible, safe, and promising for these patients, especially for patients with pseudomyxoma peritonei, as the 10-year OS of these patients was 100%.

Regarding gastric cancer peritoneal carcinomatosis treatment, there is no high-level evidence that would strongly support the use of CRS and HIPEC. Several studies from Asian countries suggested that prophylactic HIPEC in high-risk patients may improve long-term outcomes, but since they are confined to exclusively the Asian population or a small number of included patients, such treatment cannot be considered outside of clinical trials [22–25].

Taking together the current evidence, CRS with HIPEC is the cornerstone treatment option only for primary peritoneal malignancies (pseudomyxoma peritonei or malignant mesothelioma) and mucinous appendiceal tumors. Other indications, such as peritoneal metastases arising from colorectal, ovarian, and gastric cancers remain controversial. The optimization of HIPEC protocols, new drugs and techniques (i.e., water lavage), and the development and improvement of perioperative care techniques that would reduce postoperative morbidity may expand the indications for CRS with HIPEC, but further studies are needed [26–30]

The main and most important limitation of present study was its retrospective nature which greatly limited the level of evidence. This emphasizes the need for the centralization of such patients with peritoneal surface pathology, thus allowing more evidence to emerge in randomized clinical trial settings.

5. Conclusions

The current study demonstrated the results of the CRS and HIPEC program in a single Baltic country tertiary center. Patients who underwent CRS and HIPEC for PSMs achieved moderate survival rates with acceptable postoperative morbidity and mortality risk. CRS with HIPEC is a standard treatment option for primary peritoneal malignancies, and our study confirmed excellent outcomes in these patients. However, the lack of high-level evidence on CRS and HIPEC for most of the peritoneal metastases precludes the utilization of this treatment outside the clinical trial setting.

Author Contributions: R.R. contributed to data collection and analysis and was a major contributor in writing the manuscript; A.B. contributed to analyzing data and writing the manuscript; J.J. and M.P. contributed to writing and reviewing the manuscript; K.S. contributed to data analysis, manuscript writing, and the review of the manuscript. All authors have read and agreed to the published version of the manuscript.

Funding: This research received no external funding.

Institutional Review Board Statement: Vilnius regional biomedical research ethics committee approval (No. 2020/11-1279-761) was obtained before this study was conducted. The study was conducted according to the Declaration of Helsinki.

Informed Consent Statement: Informed consent was waived by the Vilnius regional biomedical research ethics committee that approved the study.

Data Availability Statement: The datasets used and/or analyzed during the current study are available from the corresponding author upon reasonable request.

Conflicts of Interest: The authors declare that they have no competing interests.

Abbreviations

PSM	primary surface malignancy
CC	completeness of cytoreduction
CRS	cytoreduction
OS	overall survival
HIPEC	hyperthermic intraperitoneal chemotherapy
LAMN	low-grade appendiceal mucinous neoplasm
HAMN	high-grade appendiceal mucinous neoplasm

References

1. Pamela, K.; Matthias, Z.; Reinhold, K.-R.; Julia, P.; Peter, M.; Alexander, P.; Dietmar, Ö. Cytoreductive Surgery (CRS) and Hyperthermic Intraperitoneal Chemotherapy (HIPEC): A Single-Center Experience in Austria. *J. Gastrointest. Surg.* **2018**, *22*, 884–893. [CrossRef]
2. Yap, D.R.Y.; Wong, J.S.M.; Tan, Q.X.; Tan, J.W.-S.; Chia, C.S.; Ong, C.-A.J. Effect of HIPEC on Peritoneal Recurrence in Peritoneal Metastasis Treated with Cytoreductive Surgery: A Systematic Review. *Front. Oncol.* **2021**, *11*, 795390. [CrossRef] [PubMed]
3. Klaver, Y.L.B.; Simkens, L.H.J.; Lemmens, V.E.P.P.; Koopman, M.; Teerenstra, S.; Bleichrodt, R.P.; De Hingh, I.H.J.T.; Punt, C.J.A. Outcomes of colorectal cancer patients with peritoneal carcinomatosis treated with chemotherapy with and without targeted therapy. *Eur. J. Surg. Oncol. (EJSO)* **2012**, *38*, 617–623. [CrossRef] [PubMed]
4. González-Moreno, S.; González-Bayón, L.A.; Ortega-Pérez, G. Hyperthermic intraperitoneal chemotherapy: Rationale and technique. *World J. Gastrointest. Oncol.* **2010**, *2*, 68. [CrossRef] [PubMed]
5. Ray, M.D.; Dhall, K. Hyperthermic Intraperitoneal Chemotherapy (HIPEC) in the management of peritoneal surface malignancies—An evidence-based review. *Curr. Probl. Cancer* **2021**, *45*, 100737. [CrossRef]
6. Quénet, F.; Elias, D.; Roca, L.; Goéré, D.; Ghouti, L.; Pocard, M.; Facy, O.; Arvieux, C.; Lorimier, G.; Pezet, D.; et al. Cytoreductive surgery plus hyperthermic intraperitoneal chemotherapy versus cytoreductive surgery alone for colorectal peritoneal metastases (PRODIGE 7): A multicentre, randomised, open-label, phase 3 trial. *Lancet Oncol.* **2021**, *22*, 256–266. [CrossRef]

7. Klaver, C.E.L.; Wisselink, D.D.; Punt, C.J.A.; Snaebjornsson, P.; Crezee, J.; Aalbers, A.G.J.; Brandt, A.; Bremers, A.J.A.; Burger, J.W.A.; Fabry, H.F.J.; et al. Adjuvant hyperthermic intraperitoneal chemotherapy in patients with locally advanced colon cancer (COLOPEC): A multicentre, open-label, randomised trial. *Lancet Gastroenterol. Hepatol.* **2019**, *4*, 761–770. [CrossRef]
8. Bonnot, P.-E.; Piessen, G.; Kepenekian, V.; Decullier, E.; Pocard, M.; Meunier, B.; Bereder, J.-M.; Abboud, K.; Marchal, F.; Quenet, F.; et al. Cytoreductive Surgery with or without Hyperthermic Intraperitoneal Chemotherapy for Gastric Cancer with Peritoneal Metastases (CYTO-CHIP study): A Propensity Score Analysis. *J. Clin. Oncol.* **2019**, *37*, 2028–2040. [CrossRef] [PubMed]
9. Moran, B.J. PROPHYLOCHIP: No benefit of second-look surgery plus HIPEC for colorectal peritoneal metastases. *Lancet Oncol.* **2020**, *21*, 1124–1125. [CrossRef]
10. Sugarbaker, P.H. New standard of care for appendiceal epithelial neoplasms and pseudomyxoma peritonei syndrome? *Lancet Oncol.* **2006**, *7*, 69–76. [CrossRef]
11. Sugarbaker, P.H. Surgical management of peritoneal carcinosis: Diagnosis, prevention and treatment. *Langenbecks Arch. Für Chir.* **1988**, *373*, 189–196. [CrossRef] [PubMed]
12. Segelman, J.; Granath, F.; Holm, T.; Machado, M.; Mahteme, H.; Martling, A. Incidence, prevalence and risk factors for peritoneal carcinomatosis from colorectal cancer. *J. Br. Surg.* **2012**, *99*, 699–705. [CrossRef] [PubMed]
13. Verwaal, V.J.; Bruin, S.; Boot, H.; Van Slooten, G.; Van Tinteren, H. 8-year follow-up of randomized trial: Cytoreduction and hyperthermic intraperitoneal chemotherapy versus systemic chemotherapy in patients with peritoneal carcinomatosis of colorectal cancer. *Ann. Surg. Oncol.* **2008**, *15*, 2426–2432. [CrossRef] [PubMed]
14. van Stein, R.M.; Aalbers, A.G.J.; Sonke, G.S.; van Driel, W.J. Hyperthermic Intraperitoneal Chemotherapy for Ovarian and Colorectal Cancer: A Review. *JAMA Oncol.* **2021**, *7*, 1231–1238. [CrossRef]
15. Lim, M.C.; Chang, S.-J.; Yoo, H.J.; Nam, B.-H.; Bristow, R.; Park, S.-Y. Randomized trial of hyperthermic intraperitoneal chemotherapy (HIPEC) in women with primary advanced peritoneal, ovarian, and tubal cancer. *J. Clin. Oncol.* **2017**, *35*, 5520. [CrossRef]
16. Ansaloni, L.; Agnoletti, V.; Amadori, A.; Catena, F.; Cavaliere, D.; Coccolini, F.; De Iaco, P.; Di Battista, M.; Framarini, M.; Gazzotti, F.; et al. Evaluation of Extensive Cytoreductive Surgery and Hyperthermic Intraperitoneal Chemotherapy (HIPEC) in Patients With Advanced Epithelial Ovarian Cancer. *Int. J. Gynecol. Cancer* **2012**, *22*, 778. [CrossRef]
17. van Driel, W.J.; Koole, S.N.; Sikorska, K.; Schagen van Leeuwen, J.H.; Schreuder, H.W.; Hermans, R.H.; De Hingh, I.H.; Van Der Velden, J.; Arts, H.J.; Massuger, L.F.; et al. Hyperthermic Intraperitoneal Chemotherapy in Ovarian Cancer. *N. Engl. J. Med.* **2018**, *378*, 230–240. [CrossRef]
18. Tsuyoshi, H.; Inoue, D.; Kurokawa, T.; Yoshida, Y. Hyperthermic intraperitoneal chemotherapy (HIPEC) for gynecological cancer. *J. Obstet. Gynaecol. Res.* **2020**, *46*, 1661–1671. [CrossRef]
19. Kusamura, S.; Barretta, F.; Yonemura, Y.; Sugarbaker, P.H.; Moran, B.J.; Levine, E.A.; Goere, D.; Baratti, D.; Nizri, E.; Morris, D.L.; et al. The Role of Hyperthermic Intraperitoneal Chemotherapy in Pseudomyxoma Peritonei after Cytoreductive Surgery. *JAMA Surg.* **2021**, *156*, e206363. [CrossRef]
20. Järvinen, P.; Ristimäki, A.; Kantonen, J.; Aronen, M.; Huuhtanen, R.; Järvinen, H.; Lepistö, A. Comparison of serial debulking and cytoreductive surgery with hyperthermic intraperitoneal chemotherapy in pseudomyxoma peritonei of appendiceal origin. *Int. J. Colorectal Dis.* **2014**, *29*, 999–1007. [CrossRef]
21. Sinukumar, S.; Mehta, S.; As, R.; Damodaran, D.; Ray, M.; Zaveri, S.; Kammar, P.; Bhatt, A. Analysis of Clinical Outcomes of Pseudomyxoma Peritonei from Appendicular Origin Following Cytoreductive Surgery and Hyperthermic Intraperitoneal Chemotherapy—A Retrospective Study from INDEPSO. *Indian J. Surg. Oncol.* **2019**, *10*, 65–70. [CrossRef] [PubMed]
22. Auer, R.C.; Sivajohanathan, D.; Biagi, J.; Conner, J.; Kennedy, E.; May, T. Indications for hyperthermic intraperitoneal chemotherapy with cytoreductive surgery: A clinical practice guideline. *Curr. Oncol.* **2020**, *27*, 146–154. [CrossRef] [PubMed]
23. Yonemura, Y.; de Aretxabala, X.; Fujimura, T.; Fushida, S.; Katayama, K.; Bandou, E.; Sugiyama, K.; Kawamura, T.; Kinoshita, K.; Endou, Y.; et al. Intraoperative chemohyperthermic peritoneal perfusion as an adjuvant to gastric cancer: Final results of a randomized controlled study. *Hepato-Gastroenterology* **2001**, *48*, 1776–1782. [PubMed]
24. Granieri, S.; Bonomi, A.; Frassini, S.; Chierici, A.P.; Bruno, F.; Paleino, S.; Kusamura, S.; Germini, A.; Facciorusso, A.; Deraco, M.; et al. Prognostic impact of cytoreductive surgery (CRS) with hyperthermic intraperitoneal chemotherapy (HIPEC) in gastric cancer patients: A meta-analysis of randomized controlled trials. *Eur. J. Surg. Oncol.* **2021**, *47*, 2757–2767. [CrossRef]
25. Seshadri, R.A.; Glehen, O. Cytoreductive surgery and hyperthermic intraperitoneal chemotherapy in gastric cancer. *World J. Gastroenterol.* **2016**, *22*, 1114–1130. [CrossRef]
26. Gasser, E.; Kogler, P.; Lorenz, A.; Kafka-Ritsch, R.; Öfner, D.; Perathoner, A. Do we still need CRS and HIPEC in colorectal cancer in times of modern chemotherapy and immunotherapy? *MEMO—Mag. Eur. Med. Oncol.* **2020**, *13*, 430–433. [CrossRef]
27. Gronau, F.; Feldbruegge, L.; Oberwittler, F.; Gonzalez-Moreno, S.; Villeneuve, L.; Eveno, C.; Glehen, O.; Kusamura, S.; Rau, B. HIPEC in Peritoneal Metastasis of Gastric Origin: A Systematic Review of Regimens and Techniques. *J. Clin. Med.* **2022**, *11*, 1456. [CrossRef] [PubMed]
28. Bijelic, L.; Crusellas, O.; Ramos, I.; Van der Speeten, K.; Barrios, P.; Sabia, D. Designing HIPEC regimens for colon cancer: Is the available evidence being appropriately considered? *Surg. Open Dig. Adv.* **2021**, *3*, 100019. [CrossRef]

29. Gabriel, E.; Singla, S.; Kim, M.; Fisher, D.; Powers, C.; Visioni, A.; Attwood, K.; Skitzki, J. Water lavage as an adjunct to cytoreductive surgery with hyperthermic intraperitoneal chemotherapy (CRS-HIPEC). *Am. J. Surg.* **2017**, *214*, 462–467. [CrossRef]
30. Almerey, T.; Gabriel, E.M.; Torp, K.D.; Bagaria, S.P. Intraoperative fluid restriction in hyperthermic intraperitoneal chemotherapy. *J. Surg. Res.* **2018**, *231*, 77–82. [CrossRef]

Journal of
Clinical Medicine

MDPI

Article

The Role of Intraperitoneal Intraoperative Chemotherapy with Paclitaxel in the Surgical Treatment of Peritoneal Carcinomatosis from Ovarian Cancer—Hyperthermia versus Normothermia: A Randomized Controlled Trial

Angela Casado-Adam [1,2], Lidia Rodriguez-Ortiz [1,2], Sebastian Rufian-Peña [1,2], Cristobal Muñoz-Casares [1,2], Teresa Caro-Cuenca [3,4], Rosa Ortega-Salas [3,4], Maria Auxiliadora Fernandez-Peralbo [5], Maria Dolores Luque-de-Castro [5], Juan M. Sanchez-Hidalgo [1,2], Cesar Hervas-Martinez [6], Antonio Romero-Ruiz [2,7], Javier Briceño [1,2] and Álvaro Arjona-Sánchez [1,2,*]

1 Oncologic and Pancreatic Surgery Unit, University Hospital Reina Sofia, Avda Menéndez Pidal s/n, 14004 Córdoba, Spain
2 CIBERehd, Maimonides Biomedical Research Institute of Cordoba (IMIBIC), University Hospital Reina Sofia, Avda Menéndez Pidal s/n, 14004 Córdoba, Spain
3 Department of Pathology, Reina Sofía University Hospital, 14004 Córdoba, Spain
4 Maimonides Biomedical Research Institute of Córdoba (IMIBIC), 14004 Córdoba, Spain
5 Department of Analytical Chemistry, Campus of Rabanales, University of Córdoba, Annex Marie Curie Building, 14071 Córdoba, Spain
6 Department of Computer Science and Numerical Analysis, University of Córdoba, 14071 Córdoba, Spain
7 Department of Biochemistry and Molecular Biology, University of Córdoba, 14004 Córdoba, Spain
* Correspondence: alvaroarjona@hotmail.com

Abstract: Background: The treatment of ovarian carcinomatosis with cytoreductive surgery and HIPEC is still controversial. The effect and pharmacokinetics of the chemotherapeutics used (especially taxanes) are currently under consideration. Methods: A phase II, simple blind and randomized controlled trial (NTC02739698) was performed. The trial included 32 patients with primary or recurrent ovarian carcinomatosis undergoing cytoreductive surgery (CRS) and intraoperative intraperitoneal chemotherapy with paclitaxel (PTX): 16 in hyperthermic (42–43 °C) and 16 in normothermic (37 °C) conditions. Tissue, serum and plasma samples were taken in every patient before and after intraperitoneal chemotherapy to measure the concentration of PTX. To analyze the immunohistochemical profile of p53, p27, p21, ki67, PCNA and caspase-3 and the pathological response, a scale of intensity and percentage of expression and a grouped Miller and Payne system were used, respectively. Perioperative characteristics and morbi-mortality were also analyzed. Results: The main characteristics of patients, surgical morbidity, hemotoxicity and nephrotoxicity were similar in both groups. The concentration of paclitaxel in the tissue was higher than that observed in plasma and serum, although no statistically significant differences were found between the two groups. No statistically significant association regarding pathological response and apoptosis (caspase-3) between both groups was proved. There were no statistically significant differences between the normothermic and the hyperthermic group for pathological response and apoptosis. Conclusions: The use of intraperitoneal PTX has proven adequate pharmacokinetics with reduction of cell cycle and proliferation markers globally without finding statistically significant differences between its administration under hyperthermia versus normothermia conditions.

Keywords: ovarian cancer; peritoneal carcinomatosis; intraperitoneal chemotherapy

1. Introduction

The standard treatment of primary advanced epithelial ovarian cancer (EOC) is complete cytoreductive surgery (CRS) with no residual tumor, followed by adjuvant chemotherapy based on taxanes and platinum compounds [1,2].

Due to its natural history, EOC remains localized in the abdominal cavity. Intraperitoneal (IP) chemotherapy allows higher concentrations of chemotherapeutics in the peritoneal cavity than systemic chemotherapy because of its slow absorption by the peritoneum and the first-pass effect by the liver. This allows higher IP doses and potentially increased efficacy with concurrently low systemic toxicity [3,4] and an increased possibility of survival. Nevertheless, this type of chemotherapy has not been fully accepted for different reasons: pharmacokinetic problems (the penetration depth of IP delivered drugs into the tumor nodules is limited [5], so optimal CRS will be required before IP chemotherapy), problems with the technique since it is not free from peritoneal access device complications with high toxicity [6] and the complex and demanding logistical management of patients. Although IP chemotherapy with taxanes has been demonstrated to be effective in advanced EOC [6], in the last GOG-252 trial no progression-free survival (PFS) improvement with IP chemotherapy was seen [7].

To overcome the inconveniences of IP chemotherapy, intraoperative administration under hyperthermia conditions (HIPEC) arose. Its main objective was to treat residual microscopic disease after CRS before the formation of adhesions, through physical (heat) and chemical (chemotherapeutic) methods [8]. The mechanisms by which HIPEC results in an increased tumor response to cytostatics, besides the direct effect of heat [9] per se, are multiple [10]. HIPEC potentiates the cytotoxic effect of some chemotherapeutic agents [11–15] and increases their tissue penetration [16,17]. There is significant heterogeneity in fundamental aspects of HIPEC administration, such as the clinical setting in which it is indicated, the definition of optimal surgery (CC1 vs. R1), the cytostatic used and its dose, the temperature (37–46 °C) or the perfusion time [18].

Some authors [19–27] (our group among them) use taxanes for HIPEC in the treatment of ovarian carcinomatosis because of its high efficacy observed in the systemic treatment of EOC and its favorable pharmacokinetics after IP administration due to its high molecular weight [28] and hepatic metabolism. The theory about an increase in the efficacy of intraperitoneal taxanes administration is supported by different clinical [29–32] and experimental studies [33,34]. In an update published by Sugarbaker [35], it was observed that hyperthermia increases the cytotoxic activity of most cytostatics. However, this synergy is not clear in taxanes. Contradictory results have been obtained concerning the interaction of heat with taxanes [36], even though they are heat stable, and hyperthermia seems to increase the intracellular accumulation of these cytostatics.

For all the above, this study aims to analyze the effect of intraoperative IP administration of paclitaxel (PTX) under hyperthermia vs. normothermia conditions on antitumor activity, proliferation and cell cycle markers and its pharmacokinetics.

2. Patients and Methods

A phase II, simple blind, randomized controlled trial (RCT), NTC02739698, was performed. All steps, including a selection of patients, sampling and storage, were developed according to the guidelines dictated by the World Medical Association Declaration of Helsinki in 2004. The ethical review board of Reina Sofía Hospital (Córdoba, Spain) approved and supervised the clinical study.

3. Inclusion Criteria

Age ranging between 18–75 years; histopathologic confirmation of peritoneal carcinomatosis from primary or recurrent EOC (stage IIIb-IIIc FIGO); Karnosfsky index > 70 or Gynecologic Oncology Group performance status $\leq$ 2; optimal or complete CRS (no residual tumor greater than 2.5 mm) and an informed consent form filled by all patients.

4. Exclusion Criteria

Unfulfillment of inclusion criteria; extra-abdominal metastasis or stage IV FIGO; concomitance of other malignant neoplasm; renal, hepatic or cardiovascular dysfunction; intolerance during treatment or refusal to participate.

5. Sample Size Calculation

Based on an expected 40% of G3 tumor-regression in the experimental arm vs. a 1% of G3 tumor-regression in the control arm with an α error of 0.05 and β error of 0.20, the sample size was 32 (16 patients per group). It has been calculated according to the available funding from the public health grant.

6. Treatment

All patients (except one) received a neoadjuvant chemotherapy regime consisting of four to six cycles of carbo-taxol. After confirming the stabilization or regression of the disease, the patients underwent optimal CRS followed by intraoperative IP chemotherapy with 60 mg/m^2 PTX per 2 l of 1.5% dextrose at continuous perfusion for 60 min. They were randomized 1:1 after the completeness of cytoreduction into two groups: the experimental arm (H-group) in which the IP chemotherapy was administered in hyperthermia conditions (41–42 °C) and the control arm (N-group) where this IP chemotherapy was administered in normothermia conditions (37 °C). After surgery, most patients received adjuvant carbo-taxol chemotherapy to complete the eight cycles.

7. Variables

Main characteristics of patients, the ovarian cancer stage, previous surgical score (PSS) [37], response to neoadjuvant chemotherapy (complete response: normalization of Ca 125 and disappearance of signs of disease in radiology tests; partial response: decrease of the value of Ca 125 and decrease of signs of disease in radiology tests according to RECIST criteria [38]) and data of surgery such as peritoneal carcinomatosis index (PCI) [39] or Completeness of Cytoreduction (CC) Score [40] were collected.

Dindo–Clavien scale [41] and CTCAE [42] v 4.0 were used to describe surgical morbidity and hematological and renal toxicities, respectively. Major morbidity was considered as $\geq$grade 3 after 30 days from the surgical treatment.

8. Sampling and Storage

Two types of peritoneal biopsies (with and without tumor) were taken before and after IP chemotherapy (PRE-chemo and POST-chemo, respectively). Those with a small and well-perfused area of infiltrated peritoneum were sent to the Pathology Department in fresh. The other tumor-free peritoneal biopsies and blood samples (taken before, immediately after and 1 h after IP chemotherapy-PRE-chemo, POST-chemo and 1 h POST-chemo, respectively), the latter after centrifugation-were introduced in Eppendorf tubes and preserved at −80 °C to analyze the concentration of PTX in peritoneal tissue by liquid chromatography-tandem mass spectrometry (LC–MS/MS), as reported before [43].

9. Anatomopathological Study

The specimens were fixed in 10% neutral formalin, routinely processed and embedded in paraffin blocks, from which 3 micrometer (µm) thick serial sections were cut and stained with HE, PAS and Masson's trichome.

The immunohistochemical study was performed using the prediluted antibodies: p53 (clone DO.7. Dako Corporation Santa Clara, CA United States), p27^{kip1} (clone DSC-72. Genova Scientific SL), p21^{waf1} (clone polyclonal. Genova Scientific SL, Seville, Spain), ki67 (clone MIB.1. Dako Corporation), PCNA (clone PC10. Genova Scientific SL, Seville, Spain) and caspase-3 (clone polyclonal. Master Diagnostica SL). For the immunostaining, the Dako EnVision Flex Plus visualization system was used. The sections were examined by two blinded expert pathologists and evaluated by the grouped Miller and Payne (MP) system [44] for pathological response: G1 (minimal changes that include MP G1-G2), G3 (microscopic foci that include MP G3-G4) and G5 (no residual tumor), according to the percentage of total area involved in the biopsy specimen. Immunohistochemical expression was assessed by the percentage of nuclei-stained tumor cells.

10. Statistical Analysis

Continuous variables were expressed as means and standard deviation (SD), and categorical variables as frequency and percentages. Association between categorical variables was tested using Pearson's chi-squared test (χ^2). The difference between means of continuous variables was tested by an independent *t*-test. The second set of dependent *t*-tests (paired samples *t*-test) was carried out to compare the means of two related groups to determine if a statistically significant difference exists between these means of anatomopathological results. p values ≤ 0.05 were defined as statistically significant.

11. Results

11.1. Patients' Main Characteristics

The main patient characteristics are presented in Table 1. No statistically significant differences in preoperative variables were found between the two groups, except BMI (24.68 ± 2.55 H-group vs. 29.00 ± 4.84 N-group, $p < 0.004$).

Table 1. Patients' main characteristics.

	H-Group (n = 16)	N-Group (n = 16)	p
Age (years)	57.06 ± 12.60	58.13 ± 9.38	0.789
BMI (kg/m^2)	24.68 ± 2.55	29.00 ± 4.84	0.004
Prior abdominal surgery			
No	13 (81.2%)	9 (56.2%)	0.253
Yes	3 (18.8%)	7 (43.8%)	
Prior comorbidity			
No	8 (50.0%)	9 (56.3%)	1
Yes	8 (50.0%)	7 (43.8%)	
Ovarian cancer situation			
Primary	15 (93.8%)	12 (75.0%)	0.33
Recurrent	1 (6.3%)	4 (25.0%)	
Prior cancer surgery			
No	10 (62.5%)	4 (25.0%)	0.075
Yes	6 (37.5%)	12 (75.0%)	
Prior Surgical Score (PSS)			
0	10 (62.5%)	4 (25.0%)	
1	4 (25.0%)	8 (50.0%)	0.164
2	2 (12.5%)	3 (28.8%)	
3	0 (0.0%)	1 (6.3%)	
Neoadjuvant chemotherapy			
No	1 (6.3%)	0 (0.0%)	0.31
Yes	15 (93.8%)	16 (100%)	
Response to neoadjuvant chemotherapy			0.714
Complete	2 (12.5%)	4 (25.0%)	
Partial	13 (81.2%)	12 (75.0%)	

H-group: Hyperthermia group, N-group: Normothermia group, BMI: Body Mass Index.

11.2. Treatment and Morbidity

The mean PCI was similar in both groups, and although microscopically complete cytoreduction (CC0) was achieved in 81.2% in H-group and 62.5% in N-group, no significant differences were found (Table 2).

Table 2. Treatment and morbidity.

	H-Group (n = 16)	N-Group (n = 16)	p
Ureteral catheterization			
No	2 (12.5%)	1 (6.3%)	0.544
Yes	14 (87.5%)	15 (93.8%)	
PCI	19.25 ± 6.78	21.50 ± 7.81	0.391
Peritonectomy procedure			
Total	11 (68.8%)	12 (75.0%)	0.462
Extensive	5 (31.3%)	3 (18.8%)	
Pelvic	0 (0.0%)	1 (6.3%)	
CC Score			
CC0	13 (81.2%)	10 (62.5%)	0.432
CC1	3 (18.8%)	6 (37.5%)	
Splenectomy			
No	12 (75.0%)	10 (62.5%)	0.703
Yes	4 (25.0%)	6 (37.5%)	
Number of anastomosis			
0	5 (31.3%)	8 (50.0%)	0.363
1	10 (62.5%)	6 (37.5%)	
2	1 (6.3%)	2 (12.5%)	
Number of procedures			
2–1	0 (0.0%)	1 (6.3%)	0.665
4–3	11 (68.8%)	10 (62.5%)	
5	5 (31.3%)	5 (31.3%)	
Intraoperative blood transfusion			
No	5 (31.3%)	9 (56.3%)	0.154
Yes	11 (68.8%)	7 (43.8%)	
Duration of surgery (minutes)	492.53 ± 95.81	538.06 ± 112.91	0.237
Postoperative blood transfusion (units)			
0	4 (25.0%)	1 (6.3%)	0.688
1–2	7 (43.8%)	7 (43.8%)	
3–4	3 (18.8%)	5 (31.3%)	
>4	2 (12.5%)	2 (12.5%)	
Postoperative stay (days)	12.38 ± 6.63	13.33 ± 6.65	0.691
Surgical Morbidity (Clavien)			
I-II	12 (75.0%)	14 (87.5%)	0.245
IIIa	3 (18.8%)	0 (0.0%)	
IIIb	1 (6.3%)	1 (6.3%)	
IVa	0 (0.0%)	1 (6.3%)	
IVb	0 (0.0%)	0 (0.0%)	
V	0 (0.0%)	0 (0.0%)	
Leukopenia (CTCAE 4.0)			
No	14 (87.5%)	15 (93.8%)	1
1	0 (0.0%)	0 (0%)	
2	0 (0.0%)	0 (0%)	
3	2 (12.5%)	1 (6.3%)	
4	0 (0.0%)	0 (0.0%)	
5	0 (0.0%)	0 (0.0%)	

Table 2. *Cont.*

	H-Group	N-Group	p
	(n = 16)	(n = 16)	
Neutropenia (CTCAE 4.0)			
No	14 (87.5%)	15 (93.8%)	
1	0 (0.0%)	0 (0.0%)	
2	0 (0.0%)	0 (0.0%)	0.491
3	1 (6.3%)	1 (6.3%)	
4	1 (6.3%)	0 (0.0%)	
5	0 (0.0%)	0 (0.0%)	
Thrombocytopenia (CTCAE 4.0)			
No	15 (93.8%)	13 (81.2%)	
1	0 (0.0%)	1 (6.3%)	
2	1 (6.3%)	2 (12.5%)	0.478
3	0 (0.0%)	0 (0.0%)	
4	0 (0.0%)	0 (0.0%)	
5	0 (0.0%)	0 (0.0%)	
Acute kidney injury (CTCAE 4.0)			
No	11 (68.8%)	6 (37.5%)	
1	2 (12.5%)	2 (12.5%)	0.346
2	1 (6.3%)	4 (25.0%)	
3	2 (12.5%)	3 (18.8%)	
4	0 (0.0%)	1 (6.3%)	
5	0 (0.0%)	0 (0.0%)	
Hematuria (CTCAE 4.0)			
No	8 (50.0%)	7 (43.5%)	
1	2 (12.5%)	2 (12.5%)	
2	6 (37.5%)	7 (43.8%)	0.931
3	0 (0.0%)	0 (0.0%)	
4	0 (0.0%)	0 (0.0%)	
5	0 (0.0%)	0 (0.0%)	

H-group: Hyperthermia group, N-group: Normothermia group, PCI: Peritoneal Carcinomatosis Index, CC score: Completeness of Cytoreduction Score, CTCAE: Common Terminology Criteria for Adverse.

There was no treatment-related death. However, all patients in this study had at least one grade 2 surgical complication since they all received total parenteral nutrition (TPN), and most patients required a blood transfusion.

Major surgical morbidity (≥ IIIa) was 25% in H-group and 12.5% in N-group. In the H-group, two patients had a wound infection that needed surgical debridement; one had low-grade colorectal fistula treated with conservative treatment and percutaneous drainage, and the other required reintervention due to hemoperitoneum. In N-group, one patient required reoperation due to hemoperitoneum, and another had septic shock with reintervention with renal and global respiratory failure, resulting in death.

Grade 3–4 hemotoxicity was seen in 9.4% (12.5% H-group vs. 6.3% N-group). Grade 3–4 nephrotoxicity was seen in 12.5% of the H-group and in 25% of the N-group (Table 2).

12. Pharmacokinetics

PRE-chemo serum, plasma and tissue samples had PTX values below the detection limit. In the H-group the mean PTX concentration in serum post-chemo and 1 h post-chemo was 16.61 ± 5.34 ng/mL and 12.18 ± 5.52 ng/mL, respectively; in plasma post-chemo and 1 h post-chemo, it was 17.24 ± 6.14 ng/mL and 11.23 ± 5.15 ng/mL, respectively; and in tissue, post-chemo, it was 1382 ± 1407.18 ng/mL. In the N-group, the mean PTX concentration in serum post-chemo and 1 h post-chemo was 14.98 ± 4.79 ng/mL and 13.37 ± 4.87 ng/mL, respectively; in plasma post-chemo and 1 h post-chemo, it was 15.14 ± 6.18 ng/mL and 12.36 ± 4.87 ng/mL, respectively; and in tissue post-chemo, it was

2093.19 ± 1777.92 ng/mL. No significant differences were found between the two groups in any measurement. However, it was observed that the concentration of PTX obtained at the local level (tissue) was much longer than the systemic (plasma and serum) in both groups (Figure 1).

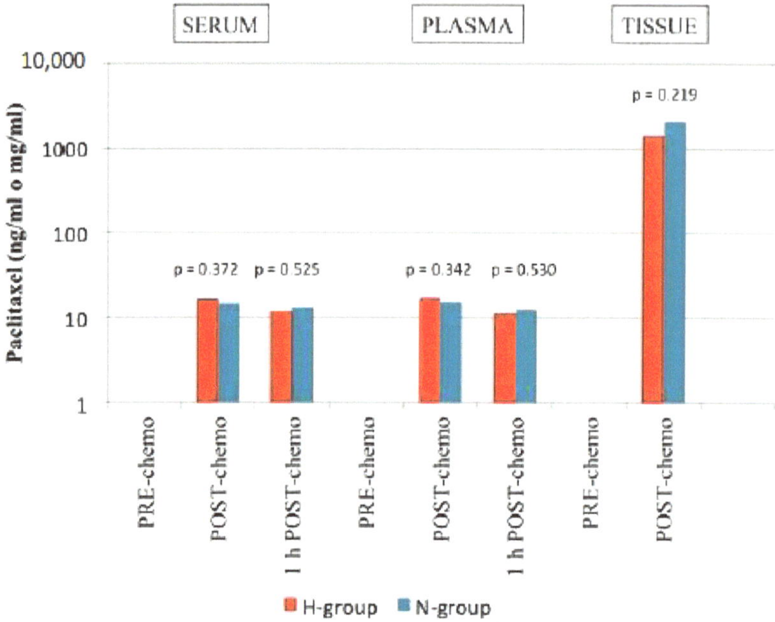

Figure 1. Pharmacokinetics of intraperitoneal PTX administration in our study. The concentration of PTX in the tissue (local level) was higher than that observed in plasma and serum (systemic level), although no statistically significant differences were found between the two groups.

13. Anatomopathology

Regarding the pathological response according to MP grouped system, no significant differences were observed in either group. It was observed that IP chemotherapy produced a marked reduction of tumor cellularity in 87.5% of the H-group and 81.3% of the N-group. The pathological reductions GR1, GR2 and GR3 were observed in 12.5%,62.5% and 25% for HIPEC group and 18.8%, 62.5% and 18.8% for the normothermic group (p = n.s) (Table 3). No significant differences concerning apoptosis (caspase-3) were found either.

The analysis of the results of the cell cycle markers (p53, p27 and p21) showed that there was a significant reduction in the expression ofW the three markers after IP chemotherapy in the 32 patients ($p = 0.021$, $p = 0.000$ and $p = 0.000$, respectively) (Figure 2), but when both groups were compared, this reduction was not statistically significant. Something similar occurred with cell proliferation markers (ki67 and PCNA). After comparing pre- and post-IP-chemo samples globally, the differences were statistically significant ($p = 0.012$ and $p = 0.000$), but not when pre- and post-chemo samples from both groups were compared (Table 3). No statistically significant differences were observed between the two groups for the cell cycle and proliferation markers.

Table 3. Anatomopathological results.

	H	N	H + N	p
	(n = 16)	(n = 16)	(n = 32)	
Pathological response				
GR1 (minimal changes)	2 (12.5%)	3 (18.8%)		0.842
GR3 (microscopic foci)	10 (62.5%)	10 (62.5%)		
GR5 (no residual tumor)	4 (25%)	3 (18.8%)		
p53				
ΔPre-Post H + N				0.021
ΔPre-Post H vs. Pre-Post N	21.56 ± 39.99	11.75 ± 37.89	16.66 ± 38.64	0.482
p27				
ΔPre-Post H + N				0
ΔPre-Post H vs. Pre-Post N	59.38 ± 38.55	44.38 ± 29.15	51.88 ± 34.47	0.224
p21				
ΔPre-Post H + N				0
ΔPre-Post H vs. Pre-Post N	36.25 ± 38.28	23.31 ± 34.02	29.78 ± 6.22	0.32
Ki67				
ΔPre-Post H + N				0.012
ΔPre-Post H vs. Pre-Post N	11.19 ± 24.32	8.88 ± 18.68	10.03 ± 21.36	0.765
PCNA				
ΔPre-Post H + N				0
ΔPre-Post H vs. Pre-Post N	47.38 ± 44.18	23.25 ± 37.49	35.31 ± 42.13	0.106
Caspasa-3				
ΔPre-Post H + N				0.188
ΔPre-Post H vs. Pre-Post N	23.44 ± 49.35	−2.81 ± 32.96	10.31 ± 43.38	0.089

H: hyperthermia, N: normothermia.

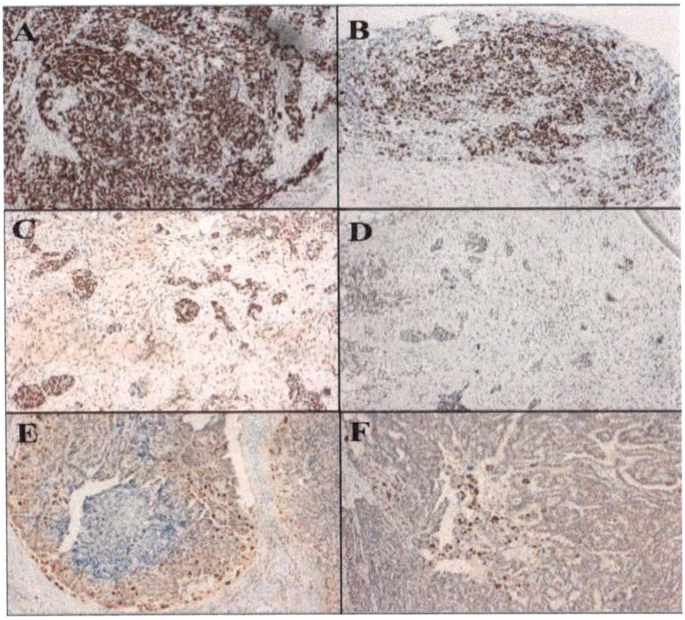

Figure 2. Immunohistochemical nuclear expression of cell cycle regulatory proteins in one H-group patient. In the analysis of the expression of the cell cycle regulatory proteins (p53, p21 and p27) in this patient, it is observed that in the pre-chemo samples the positive nuclear labeling (brown staining) is much more abundant than in the samples post-chemo; that is, there is a significant reduction in its expression after chemotherapy. (**A**): p53 pre-chemo, (**B**): p53 post-chemo, (**C**): p27 pre-chemo, (**D**): p27 post-chemo, (**E**): p21 pre-chemo, (**F**): p21 post-chemo.

14. Discussion

The present study has not shown statistically significant differences in regression grade, pharmacokinetic or molecular markers when the PTX was administered intraperitoneally in normothermia vs. hypethermia conditions. However, our study found that PTX is an excellent drug to be used intraperitoneally independent of hyperthermia conditions.

Numerous worldwide medical centers have incorporated CRS with peritonectomy procedures associated to HIPEC to treat peritoneal carcinomatosis, making this technique controversial when the carcinomatosis originates from the colon [45,46]; however, nowadays such treatment is the standard care in pseudomyxoma peritonei [47,48] and mesothelioma [49]. Although the standard treatment of ovarian carcinomatosis is not CRS-HIPEC [1,2], evidence of its use is growing after recent publications of RCTs [50–53] and meta-analyses [54,55].

Spiliotis et al. [50] reported an improvement in survival in the treatment of recurrent EOC with CRS-HIPEC vs. CRS alone, where the mean overall survival (OS) was 26.7 vs. 13.4 months respectively. However, this study has limitations considering the randomization process and the definition of the end points, which affect the interpretation of the results [56]. Moreover, others [57,58] have raised the concern that the statistical analysis performed in the study was not clearly described and inappropriately applied and their recalculation of statistics demonstrated no statistically significant differences between the two groups.

For primary EOC, better disease-free survival (DFS) rates and OS were observed in patients treated with neoadjuvant chemotherapy (NAC) followed by interval CRS-HIPEC, compared to those treated with NAC followed by interval CRS alone [51–53].

The first meta-analysis [54] of CRS-HIPEC in EOC concludes that this combination improves OS rates for both primary and recurrent EOC vs. isolated CRS. However, this meta-analysis did not provide the exact pooled hazard ratios associated with HIPEC in the clinical setting. A later meta-analysis [55] concluded, for primary EOC, that CRS-HIPEC improved both DFS and OS (in patients with a residual tumor $\leq$ 1 cm, while not visible tumors improved DFS but not OS). In case of recurrent EOC, CRS-HIPEC improved OS but not DFS (in patients with residual tumor $\leq$ 1 cm or not visible tumor improved DFS, while in patients with residual tumor $\leq$ 1 cm only improved OS).

Our group has carried out the CRS-HIPEC with PTX in the treatment of ovarian carcinomatosis since 1997 [59]. However, in the beginning, it was not always possible to use the perfusion machine that allowed reaching hyperthermia, and IP chemotherapy was administered in normothermia conditions observing how these patients reached similar conditions of survival. This behavior, added to the contradictory results obtained concerning the interaction of heat with taxanes [35], led us to decide to perform the present study.

The analysis of the results showed two homogeneous groups according to pre- and peri-operatives variables, except BMI, which was significantly higher in the N-group. However, this difference did not affect either group's ability to achieve optimal cytoreduction, which is consistent with the literature as well [60]. The morbidity and mortality outcomes of CRS-HIPEC were similar to the literature [61,62], with the total significant morbidity of 25% in the H-group and 12.5% in the N-group. Although twice as much, no significant differences were found between the two groups. Major morbidity related to intraperitoneal PTX, such as hematological and renal toxicity, ranged from 10.5% to 84.2% and 0% to 7%, respectively [6,63,64]. For HIPEC PTX administration, the major hematological toxicity is reported from 0% to 13% [22,65] and renal toxicity above 11,6% [66]. In our study, we observed significant hematological complications in 12.5% of the H-group and 6.3% of the N-group and major renal toxicity in 12.5% of the H-group and 25% of the N-group, which were not statistically different.

In our study, the maximal tissue concentrations were average, 84.54 and 178.01 times longer than the maximal plasma concentration (H and N-group, respectively). This fact supports the idea that PTX could be suitable for IP administration, according to previous reports of intraperitoneal use of PTX [22,67]. Although PTX concentration in the N-group was almost twice that of H-group, this fact might be related to the contradictory results of the effect of hyperthermia on the pharmacokinetics of taxanes [36], and no significant differences were observed in both groups.

To assess the effect of IP administration of PTX on the pathological response (reduction in tumor cellularity) we used the grouped Miller and Payne system, widely studied in the effect of neoadjuvant on locally advanced breast cancer [68] but not used previously in the treatment of ovarian cancer with HIPEC. Although we did not find significant differences in our study in the two groups, it was observed that IP chemotherapy produced a marked reduction of tumor cellularity in 87.5% of the H-group and 81.3% of the N-group.

Proliferation and cell cycle control are central processes in the biology of cancer [69], and our study showed for the first time the effect of HIPEC on these biomarkers. As p53 mutation seems to be related to the development of chemoresistance and recurrence [70,71], the relevance of the expression p21 and p27 as prognostic survival factors in EOC are inconsistent [72–75]. Our findings showed a reduction in the expression of the three markers after IP chemotherapy in both groups, but no statistically significant differences were found among them. That shows the possible influence of IP chemotherapy in the molecular field of EOC. More studies are needed to assess these findings. In an experimental setting, the hyperthermia with IP PTX used in mice with EOC enhanced the antitumor effects through immune-mediated cancer stem cell targeting [76]. In an experimental study from De Bree et al. [77], the absence of thermal enhancement (the normothermic), as our study showed, may be as effective as hyperthermic intraoperative intraperitoneal chemotherapy with taxanes. Potential oncological and treatment-related adverse effects of concurrent hyperthermia, such as thermal injury to organs and other tissues [78], immunosuppressive effects [79] and the enhanced systemic release of heat-shock proteins [80–82], could be avoided.

The main limitation of this study is the small sample size, even though our hospital is a reference for the treatment of ovarian carcinomatosis in our country, so it will be necessary to conduct additional studies with a larger sample size to validate the impact of the temperature in IP administration of PTX on pharmacokinetics, pathological response and cell cycle markers. Nevertheless, to our knowledge, this is the first study in ovarian carcinomatosis where IP chemotherapy is compared with taxanes in hyperthermia vs. normothermia conditions.

In conclusion, in this clinical trial, PTX has proven to have adequate pharmacokinetics to treat ovarian carcinomatosis, reaching optimal concentrations in tissue and minimal in serum and plasma, as well as a reduction in cell cycle and proliferation markers globally when administered in the peritoneal cavity during CRS. Nevertheless, no significant differences in pharmacokinetics and cytotoxicity could be demonstrated between normothermic and hyperthermic intraoperative intraperitoneal chemotherapy in patients with primary or recurrent ovarian cancer.

Author Contributions: Data curation, S.R.-P. and T.C.-C.; Formal analysis, R.O.-S., M.A.F.-P., M.D.L.-d.-C., J.M.S.-H., C.H.-M. and A.R.-R.; Investigation, C.M.-C. and Á.A.-S.; Methodology, A.C.-A. and J.B.; Project administration, L.R.-O. All authors have read and agreed to the published version of the manuscript.

Funding: This research was supported by "Aid Biomedical Research and Health Sciences in Andalucia" and by The Public Foundation Progress and Health Andalusian, Health Counseling, Junta de Andalucia. PI 0678-10. N° EudraCT: 2011-004373-89. ClinicalTrial.gov Identifier: NCT02739698.

Institutional Review Board Statement: The ethical review board of Reina Sofía Hospital (Córdoba, Spain) approved and supervised the clinical study. Complejo Hospitalario Regional Reina Sofia. Code: PI 0678-10, 29 December 2011.

Informed Consent Statement: Informed consent form is filled by all patients.

Data Availability Statement: Data available contacting with first or corresponding authors previously.

Acknowledgments: All staff who have participated directly or indirectly in the realization of this study, especially the Department of Analytical Chemistry of the University of Córdoba, the Department of Pathology and the Oncologic and Pancreatic Surgery Unit of Reina Sofia Hospital, are thanked.

Conflicts of Interest: There are no conflict of interest in the work submitted among the participating authors.

References

1. National Comprehensive Cancer Network. NCCN Clinical Practice Guidelines in Oncology: Ovarian Cancer including Fallopian Tube Cancer and Primary Peritoneal Cancer. V. 1.2016. Available online: https://www.tri-kobe.org/nccn/guideline/gynecological/english/ovarian.pdf (accessed on 1 March 2017).
2. Gonzalez-Martín, A.; Bover, I.; Del Campo, J.M.; Redondo, A.; Vidal, L.; Oncology, S.S.F.M. SEOM guideline in ovarian cancer 2014. *Clin. Transl. Oncol.* **2014**, *16*, 1067–1071. [CrossRef]
3. Dedrick, R.L.; Myers, C.E.; Bungay, P.M.; DeVita, V.T. Pharmacokinetic rationale for peritoneal drug administration in the treatment of ovarian cancer. *Cancer Treat. Rep.* **1978**, *62*, 1–11.
4. Markman, M. Intraperitoneal chemotherapy. *Semin. Oncol.* **1991**, *18*, 248–254.
5. Dedrick, R.L.; Flessner, M.F. Pharmacokinetic problems in peritoneal drug administration: Tissue penetration and surface exposure. *J. Natl. Cancer Inst.* **1997**, *89*, 480–487. [CrossRef]
6. Armstrong, D.K.; Bundy, B.; Wenzel, L.; Huang, H.Q.; Baergen, R.; Lele, S.; Copeland, L.J.; Walker, J.L.; Burger, R.A. Intraperitoneal cisplatin and paclitaxel in ovarian cancer. *N. Engl. J. Med.* **2006**, *354*, 34–43. [CrossRef]
7. Walker, J.L.; Brady, M.F.; Wenzel, L.; Fleming, G.F.; Huang, H.Q.; DiSilvestro, P.A.; Fujiwara, K.; Alberts, D.S.; Zheng, W.; Tewari, K.S.; et al. Randomized trial of intravenous versus intraperitoneal chemotherapy plus bevacizumab in advanced ovarian carcinoma: An NRG Oncology/Gynecologic Oncology Group Study. *J. Clin. Oncol.* **2019**, *37*, 1380–1390. [CrossRef] [PubMed]
8. Sugarbaker, P.H. It´s what the surgeon doesn´t see that kills the patient. *J. Nippon. Med. Sch.* **2000**, *67*, 5–8. [CrossRef]
9. De Bree, E.; Romanos, J.; Tsiftsis, D.D. Hyperthermia in anticancer treatment. *Eur. J. Surg. Oncol.* **2002**, *28*, 95. [CrossRef]
10. Barrasa, A.; Van de Speeten, K.; Anthony Stuart, O.; Hendrick Sugarbaker, P.; Zappa, L. Rationale for perioperative chemotherapy treatment in peritoneal carcinomatosis. *Cirugía Española* **2009**, *85*, 3–13. [CrossRef]
11. Hahn, G.M.; Braun, J.; Har-Kedar, I. Thermochemotherapy: Synergism between hyperthermia (42–43 degrees) and adriamycin (of bleomycin) in mammalian cell inactivation. *Proc. Natl. Acad. Sci. USA* **1975**, *72*, 937–940. [CrossRef]
12. Van Ruth, S.; Mathot, R.A.; Sparidans, R.W.; Beijnen, J.H.; Verwaal, V.J.; Zoetmulder, F.A. Population pharmacokinetics and pharmacodynamics of mitomycin during intraoperative hyperthermic intraperitoneal chemotherapy. *Clin. Pharmacokinet.* **2004**, *43*, 131–143. [CrossRef] [PubMed]
13. Kusumoto, T.; Holden, S.A.; Ara, G.; Teicher, B.A. Hyperthermia and platinum complexes: Time betwwen treatments and synergy in vitro and in vivo. *Int. J. Hyperth.* **1995**, *11*, 575–586. [CrossRef] [PubMed]
14. Urano, M.; Ling, C.C. Thermal enhancement of melphalan and oxaliplatin cytotoxicity in vitro. *Int. J. Hyperth.* **2002**, *18*, 307–315. [CrossRef] [PubMed]
15. Mohamed, F.; Marchettini, P.; Stuart, O.A.; Urano, M.; Sugarbaker, P.H. Thermal enhancement of new chemotherapeutic agents at moderate hyperthermia. *Ann. Surg. Oncol.* **2003**, *10*, 463–468. [CrossRef]
16. Benoit, L.; Duvillard, C.; Rat, P.; Chauffert, B. Effects de la temperature intra-abdominale sur la difusion tissulaire et tumorale du cisplatine intrapéritonéal dans un modèle de carcinose péritonéale chez le rat. *Chirurgie* **1999**, *124*, 375–379. [CrossRef]
17. Jacquet, P.; Averbach, A.; Stuart, O.A.; Chang, D.; Sugarbaker, P.H. Hyperthermic intraperitoneal doxorrubicin: Pharmacokinetics, metabolism, and tissue distribution in a rat model. *Cancer Chemother. Pharmacol.* **1998**, *41*, 147–154. [CrossRef]
18. Cascales, P.A.; Gil, J.; Galindo, P.J.; Machado, F.; Frutos, I.M.; Paricio, P.P. Heteronegecity in patients and methods. A problem for hyperthermic intraoperative intraperitoneal chemotherapy (HIPEC) in ovarian carcinoma. *Eur. J. Obstet. Gynecol. Reprod. Biol.* **2011**, *158*, 361–362. [CrossRef]
19. De Bree, E.; Romanos, J.; Michalakis, J.; Relakis, K.; Georgoulias, V.; Melissas, J.; Tsifsis, D.D. Intraoperative hyperthermic intraperitoneal chemotherapy with docetaxel as second-line treatment for peritoneal carcinomatosis of gynaecological origin. *Anticancer Res.* **2003**, *23*, 3019–3027.
20. Rufián, S.; Muñoz-Casares, F.C.; Briceño, J.; Díaz, C.J.; Rubio, M.J.; Ortega, R.; Ciria, R.; Morillo, M.; Aranda, E.; Muntané, J.; et al. Radical surgery-peritonectomy and intraoperative intraperitoneal chemotherapy for the treatment of peritoneal carcinomatosis in recurrent or primary ovarian cancer. *J. Surg. Oncol.* **2006**, *94*, 316–324. [CrossRef]
21. Bae, J.H.; Lee, J.M.; Ryu, K.S.; Lee, Y.S.; Park, Y.G.; Hur, S.Y.; Ahn, W.S.; Namkoong, S.E. Treatment of ovarian cancer with paclitaxel or carboplatin based intraperitoneal hyperthermic chemotherapy during secondary surgery. *Gynecol. Oncol.* **2007**, *106*, 193–200. [CrossRef]
22. De Bree, E.; Rosing, H.; Filis, D.; Romanos, J.; Melisssourgaki, M.; Daskalakis, M.; Pilatou, M.; Sanidas, E.; Taflampas, P.; Kalbakis, K.; et al. Cytoreductive surgery and intraoperative hyperthermic intraperitoneal chemotherapy with paclitaxel: A clinical and pharmacokinetic study. *Ann. Surg. Oncol.* **2008**, *15*, 83–92. [CrossRef]

23. Muñoz-Casares, F.C.; Rufián, S.; Rubio, M.J.; Díaz, C.J.; Díaz, R.; Casado, A.; Muñoz-Villanueva, M.C.; Muntané, J. The role of hyperthermic intraoperative intraperitoneal chemotherapy (HIPEC) in the treatment of peritoneal carcinomatosis in recurrent ovarian cancer. *Clin. Transl. Oncol.* **2009**, *11*, 753–759. [CrossRef]
24. Kim, J.H.; Lee, J.M.; Ryu, K.S.; Lee, Y.S.; Park, Y.G.; Hur, S.Y.; Lee, K.H.; Lee, S.H.; Kim, S.J. Consolidation hyperthermic intraperitoneal chemotherapy using paclitaxel in patients with epithelial ovarian cancer. *J. Surg. Oncol.* **2010**, *101*, 149–155. [CrossRef]
25. Ansaloni, L.; Agnoletti, V.; Amadori, A.; Catena, F.; Cavaliere, D.; Coccolini, F.; De Iaco, P.; Di Battista, M.; Framarini, M.; Gazzotti, F.; et al. Evaluation of extensive cytoreductive surgery and hyperthermic intraperitoneal chemotherapy (HIPEC) in patients with advanced epithelial ovarian cancer. *Int. J. Gynecol. Cancer* **2012**, *22*, 778–785. [CrossRef]
26. Cascales-Campos, P.A.; Gil, J.; Gil, E.; Feliciangeli, E.; González-Gil, A.; Parrilla, J.J.; Parrilla, P. Treatment of microscopic disease with hyperthermic intraoperative intraperitoneal chemotherapy after complete cytoreduction improves disease-free survival in patients with stage IIIC/IV ovarian cancer. *Ann. Surg. Oncol.* **2014**, *21*, 2383–2389. [CrossRef]
27. Muñoz-Casares, F.; Fernández, F.J.M.; Arjona-Sánchez, Á.; Casado-Adam, J.M.; Hidalgo, J.M.S.; Rubio, M.; Ortega-Salas, R.; Muñoz-Villanueva, M.; Rufián-Peña, S.; Briceño, F. Peritonectomy procedures and HIPEC in the treatment of peritoneal carcinomatosis from ovarian cancer: Long-term outcomes and perspectives from a high-volume center. *Eur. J. Surg. Oncol.* **2016**, *42*, 224–233. [CrossRef]
28. Sugarbaker, P.H. *An Overview of Peritonectomy, Visceral Resections, and Perioperative Chemotherapy for Peritoneal Surface Malignancy: Texbook and Video Atlas*; Ciné-Med Publishing: Woodbury, CT, USA, 2013; ISBN 978-0-9846171-5-9.
29. Kohn, E.C.; Sarosy, G.; Bicher, A.; Link, C.; Christian, M.; Steinberg, S.M.; Rothenberg, M.; Adamo, D.O.; Davis, P.; Ognibene, F.P.; et al. Dose-intense taxol: High response rate in patients with platinum-resistant recurrent ovarian cancer. *J. Natl. Cancer Inst.* **1994**, *86*, 18–24. [CrossRef]
30. Omura, G.A.; Brady, M.F.; Look, K.Y.; Averette, H.E.; Delmore, J.E.; Long, H.J.; Wadler, S.; Spiegel, G.; Arbuck, S.G. Phase III trial of paclitaxel at two dose levels, the higher dose accompanies by filgrastim at two dose levels in platinum pretreated epithelial ovarian cancer: An intergroup study. *J. Clin. Oncol.* **2003**, *21*, 2843–2848. [CrossRef]
31. Reed, E.; Bitton, R.; Sarosy, G. Paclitaxel dose intensity. *J. Infus. Chemother.* **1996**, *6*, 59–63.
32. Takimoto, C.H.; Rowinsky, E.K. Dose-intense paclitaxel: Déjà vu all over again? *J. Clin. Oncol.* **2003**, *21*, 2810–2814. [CrossRef]
33. Michalakis, J.; Georgatos, S.D.; de Bree, E.; Polioudaki, H.; Romanos, J.; Georgoulias, V.; Tsiftsis, D.D.; Theodoropoulos, P.A. Short term exposure of cancer cells to micromolar doses of paclitaxel, with or without hyperthermia, induces long term inhibition of cell proliferation and cell death in vitro. *Ann. Surg. Oncol.* **2007**, *14*, 1220–1228. [CrossRef]
34. Michalakis, J.; Georgatos, S.D.; Romanos, J.; Koutala, H.; Georgoulias, V.; Tsiftsis, D.; Theodoropoulos, P.A. Micromolar taxol, with or withou hyperthermia, induces mitotic catastrophe and cell necrosis in HeLa cells. *Cancer Chemother. Pharmacol.* **2005**, *56*, 615–622. [CrossRef]
35. Sugarbaker, P.H.; Mora, J.T.; Carmignani, P.; Stuart, O.A.; Yoo, D. Update on chemotherapeutic agents utilized for perioperative intraperitoneal chemotherapy. *Oncologist* **2005**, *10*, 112–122. [CrossRef]
36. De Bree, E.; Theodoropoulos, P.A.; Rosing, H.; Michalakis, J.; Romanos, J.; Beijnen, J.H.; Tsifsis, D.D. Treatment of ovarian cancer using intraperitoneal chemotherapy with taxanes: From laboratory bench to bedside. *Cancer Treat. Rev.* **2006**, *32*, 471–482. [CrossRef] [PubMed]
37. Jacquet, P.; Sugarbaker, P.H. Current methologies for clinical assessment of patients with peritoneal carcinomatosis. *J. Exp. Clin. Cancer Res.* **1996**, *15*, 46–58.
38. Therasse, P.; Arbuck, S.G.; Eisenhauer, E.A.; Wanders, J.; Kaplan, R.S.; Rubinstein, L.; Verweij, J.; Van Glabbeke, M.; Van Oosterom, A.T.; Christian, M.C.; et al. New guidelines to evaluate the response to treatment in solid tumors. *J. Natl. Cancer Inst.* **2000**, *92*, 205–216. [CrossRef]
39. Jacquet, P.; Sugarbaker, P.H. Clinical research methodologies in diagnosis and staging of patients with peritoneal carcinomatosis. *Cancer Treat. Res.* **1996**, *82*, 359–374.
40. Sugarbaker, P.H. Peritonectomy procedure. *Ann. Surg.* **1995**, *221*, 29–42. [CrossRef]
41. Dindo, D.; Demartines, N.; Clavien, P.A. Clasification of surgical complications. A new proposal with evaluation in a cohort of 6336 patients and results of a survey. *Ann. Surg.* **2004**, *240*, 205–213. [CrossRef]
42. National Cancer Institute (NCI); National Institutes of Health (NIH). Common Terminology Criteria for Adverse Events (CTCAE). Version 4.0 Published: 28 May 2009 (v4.03: 14 June 2010). Available online: https://evs.nci.nih.gov/ftp1/CTCAE/CTCAE_4.03_2010-06-14_QuickReference_5x7.pdf (accessed on 5 March 2011).
43. Fernández-Peralbo, M.A.; Priego-Capote, F.; Luque de Castro, M.D.; Casado-Adam, A.; Arjona-Sánchez, A.; Muñoz-Casares, F.C. LC–MS/MS quantitative analysis of paclitaxel and its major metabolites in serum, plasma and tissue from women with ovarian cancer after intraperitoneal chemoterapy. *J. Pharm. Biomed. Anal.* **2014**, *91*, 131–137. [CrossRef]
44. Ogston, K.N.; Miller, I.D.; Payne, S.; Hutcheon, A.W.; Sarkar, T.K.; Smith, I.; Schofield, A.; Heys, S.D. A new histological grading system to assess response of breast cancers to primary chemotherapy: Prognostic significance and survival. *Breast* **2003**, *12*, 320–327. [CrossRef]
45. Yan, T.D.; Black, D.; Savady, R.; Sugarbaker, P.H. Systematic review on the efficacy of cytoreductive surgey combined with perioperative intraperitoneal chemotherapy for peritoneal carcinomatosis from colorectal carcinoma. *J. Clin. Oncol.* **2006**, *24*, 4011–4019. [CrossRef] [PubMed]

46. Cao, C.; Yan, T.D.; Black, D.; Morris, D.L. A systematic review and meta-anaysis of cytoreductive surgery with perioperative intraperitoneal chemotherapy for peritoneal carcinomatosis of colorectal origin. *Ann. Surg. Oncol.* **2009**, *16*, 2152–2162. [CrossRef] [PubMed]
47. Moran, B.; Baratti, D.; Yan, T.D.; Kusamura, S.; Deraco, M. Consensus statement on the loco-regional treatment of appendiceal mucinous neoplasms with peritoneal dissemination (pseudomyxoma peritonei). *J. Surg. Oncol.* **2008**, *98*, 277–282. [CrossRef] [PubMed]
48. Chua, T.C.; Moran, B.J.; Sugarbaker, P.H.; Levine, E.A.; Glehen, O.; Gilly, F.N.; Elias, D.; Baratti, D.; Deraco, M.; Sardi, A.; et al. Early and long-term outcome data of 2298 patients with pseudomyxoma peritonei of appendiceal origin treated by a stratey of cytoreductive surgery and hyperthermic intraperitoneal chemotherapy. *J. Clin. Oncol.* **2012**, *30*, 2449–2456. [CrossRef] [PubMed]
49. Yan, T.D.; Deraco, M.; Baratti, D.; Kusamura, S.; Elias, D.; Glehen, O.; Gilly, F.N.; Levine, E.A.; Shen, P.; Mohamed, F.; et al. Cytoreductive surgery and hyperthermic intraperitoneal chemotherapy for malignat peritoneal mesothelioma: Multi-institutional experience. *J. Surg. Oncol.* **2009**, *27*, 6237–6242. [CrossRef]
50. Spiliotis, J.; Halkia, E.; Lianos, E.; Kalantzi, N.; Grivas, A.; Efstathiou, E.; Giassas, S. Cytoreductive surgery and HIPEC in recurrent epitelial ovarian cancer: A prospective randomized phase III study. *Ann. Surg. Oncol.* **2015**, *22*, 1570–1575. [CrossRef]
51. Van Driel, W.J.; Koole, S.N.; Sikorska, K.; Schagen van Leeuwen, J.H.; Schreuder, H.W.R.; Hermans, R.H.M.; De Hingh, I.H.; Van Der Velden, J.; Arts, H.J.; Massuger, L.F.; et al. Hyperthermic Intraperitoneal Chemotherapy in Ovarian Cancer. *N. Engl. J. Med.* **2018**, *378*, 230–240. [CrossRef]
52. Antonio, C.C.P.; Gil Alida, G.; Elena, G.G.; Rocío, G.S.; Jerónimo, M.G.; Luis, A.R.J.; Aníbal, N.D.; Francisco, B.V.; Jesús, G.R.; Pablo, R.R.; et al. Cytoreductive Surgery with or without HIPEC after Neoadjuvant Chemotherapy in Ovarian Cancer: A Phase 3 Clinical Trial. *Ann. Surg. Oncol.* **2022**, *29*, 2617–2625. [CrossRef]
53. Lim, M.C.; Chang, S.-J.; Park, B.; Yoo, H.J.; Yoo, C.W.; Nam, B.H.; Park, S.-Y.; Seo, S.-S.; Kang, S.; Yun, J.Y.; et al. Survival After Hyperthermic Intraperitoneal Chemotherapy and Primary or Interval Cytoreductive Surgery in Ovarian Cancer: A Randomized Clinical Trial. *JAMA Surg.* **2022**, *157*, 374–383. [CrossRef]
54. Huo, Y.R.; Richards, A.; Liauw, W.; Morris, D.L. Hyperthermic intraperitoneal chemotherapy (HIPEC) and cytoreductive surgery (CRS) in ovarian cancer: A systematic review and meta-analysis. *Eur. J. Surg. Oncol.* **2015**, *41*, 1578–1589. [CrossRef] [PubMed]
55. Kim, S.I.; Cho, J.; Lee, E.J.; Park, S.; Park, S.J.; Seol, A.; Lee, N.; Yim, G.W.; Lee, M.; Lim, W.; et al. Selection of patients with ovarian cancer who may show survival benefit from hyperthermic intraperitoneal chemotherapy: A systematic review and meta-analysis. *Medicine* **2019**, *98*, e18355. [CrossRef] [PubMed]
56. Harter, P.; Reuss, A.; Sehouli, J.; Chiva, L.; du Bois, A. Brief report about the role of hyperthermic intraperitoneal chemotherapy in a prospective randomized phase 3 study in recurrent ovarian cancer from Spiliotis et al. *Int. J. Gynecol. Cancer.* **2017**, *27*, 246–247. [CrossRef] [PubMed]
57. Batista, T.P. Comment on: Surgery and HIPEC in recurrent epithelial ovarian cancer: A prospective randomized phase III study. *Ann. Surg. Oncol.* **2017**, *24* (Suppl. 3), 630. [CrossRef] [PubMed]
58. Sanz Rubiales, Á.; Del Valle, M.L. Survival analysis in a randomized trial of HIPEC in ovarian cancer. *Ann. Surg. Oncol.* **2017**, *24* (Suppl. 3), 631. [CrossRef] [PubMed]
59. Arjona-Sánchez, A.; Rufián-Peña, S. Progress in the management of primary and recurrent ovarian carcinomatosis with peritonectomy procedures and HIPEC in a high volumen center. *Int. J. Hyperth.* **2017**, *33*, 554–561. [CrossRef] [PubMed]
60. Fotopoulou, C.; Richter, R.; Braicu, E.-I.; Kuhberg, M.; Feldheiser, A.; Schefold, J.C.; Lichtenegger, W.; Sehouli, J. Impact of obesity on operative morbidiy and clinical outcome in primary epithelial ovarian cancer after optimal primary tumor debulking. *Ann. Surg. Oncol.* **2011**, *18*, 2629–2637. [CrossRef]
61. Backes, F.J.; Nagel, C.I.; Bussewitz Donner, J.; Hade, E.; Salani, R. The impact of body weight on ovarian cancer outcomes. *Int. J. Gynecol. Cancer* **2011**, *21*, 1601–1605. [CrossRef]
62. Chua, T.C.; Yan, T.D.; Saxena, A.; Morris, D.L. Should the treatment of peritoneal carcinomatosis by cytoreductive surgery and hyperthermic intraperitoneal chemotherapy still be regarded as a highly morbid prodecure?: A systematic review of morbidity and mortality. *Ann. Surg.* **2009**, *249*, 900–907. [CrossRef]
63. Canda, A.E.; Sokmen, S.; Terzi, C.; Arslan, C.; Oztop, I.; Karabulut, B.; Ozzeybek, D.; Sarioglu, S.; Fuzun, M. Complications and toxicities after cytoreductive surgery and hyperthermic intraperitoneal chemotherapy. *Ann. Surg. Oncol.* **2013**, *20*, 1082–1087. [CrossRef]
64. Kim, S.W.; Paek, J.; Nam, E.J.; Kim, S.H.; Kim, J.H.; Kim, Y.T. The feasibility of carboplatin-based intraperitoneal chemotherapy in ovarian cancer. *Eur. J. Obstet. Gynecol. Reprod. Biol.* **2010**, *152*, 195–199. [CrossRef] [PubMed]
65. Cascales Campos, P.; Gil, J.; Parrilla, P. Morbidity and mortality outcomes of cytoreductive surgery and hypertehrmic intraperitoneal chemotherapy in patients with primary and recurrent advanced ovarian cancer. *Eur J. Surg. Oncol.* **2014**, *40*, 970–975. [CrossRef] [PubMed]
66. Arjona-Sánchez, A.; Cadenas-Febres, A.; Cabrera-Bermon, J.; Muñoz-Casares, F.; Casado-Adam, A.; Sánchez-Hidalgo, J.; López-Andreu, M.; Briceño-Delgado, J.; Rufián-Peña, S. Assesment of RIFLE and AKIN criteria to define acute renal disease for HIPEC procedures for ovarian and non ovarian peritoneal malignances. *Eur. J. Surg. Oncol.* **2016**, *42*, 869–876. [CrossRef]
67. Ansaloni, L.; Coccolini, F.; Morosi, L.; Ballerini, A.; Ceresoli, M.; Grosso, G.; Bertoli, P.L.; Busci, L.; Lotti, M.; Cambria, F.; et al. Pharmacokinetics of concomitant cisplatin and paclitaxel administered by hyperthermic intraperitoneal chemotherapy top atientes with peritoneal cacinomatosis from epithelial ovarian cancer. *Br. J. Cancer* **2015**, *112*, 306–312. [CrossRef] [PubMed]
68. Shintia, C.; Endang, H.; Diani, K. Assessment of pathological response to neoadjuvant chemotherapy in locally advanced breast cancer using the Miller-Payne system and TUNEL. *Malays. J. Pathol.* **2016**, *38*, 25–32. [PubMed]

69. Belt, E.J.T.; Brosens, R.P.M.; Diemen, P.M.D.-V.; Bril, H.; Tijssen, M.; Van Essen, D.F.; Heymans, M.; Beliën, J.A.M.; Stockmann, H.B.A.C.; Meijer, S.; et al. Cell cycle proteins predict recurrence in stage II and III colon cancer. *Ann. Surg. Oncol.* **2012**, *19* (Suppl. 3), S682–S692. [CrossRef]
70. Vang, R.; Levine, D.A.; Soslow, R.A.; Zaloudek, C.; Shih, I.e.M.; Kurman, R.J. Molecular alterations of PT53 are a defining feature of ovarian high-grade serous carcinoma: A rereview of cases lacking TP53 mutations in the Cancer Genome Atlas ovarian study. *Int. J. Gynecol. Pathol.* **2016**, *35*, 48–55. [CrossRef]
71. Zhang, M.; Zhuang, G.; Sun, X.; Shen, Y.; Wang, W.; Li, Q.; Di, W. TP53 mutation-mediated genomic instability induces the evolution of chemoresistance and recurrence in epitelial ovarian cancer. *Diagn. Pathol.* **2017**, *12*, 16. [CrossRef]
72. Skirnisdottir, I.; Seidal, T. Association of p21, p21 p27 and p21 p53 status to histological subtypes and prognosis in low-stage epithelial ovarian cancer. *Cancer Genom. Proteom.* **2013**, *10*, 27–34.
73. Geisler, H.E.; Geisler, J.P.; Miller, G.A.; Geisler, M.J.; Wiemann, M.C.; Zhou, Z.; Crabtree, W. p21 and p53 in ovarian carcinoma: Their combined staining is more valuable than their alone. *Cancer* **2001**, *92*, 781–786. [CrossRef]
74. Schmider-Ross, A.; Pirsig, O.; Gottschalk, E.; Denkert, C.; Lichtenegger, W.; Reles, A. Cyclin-dependent kinase inhibitors CIP1(p21) and KIP1 (p27) in ovarian cancer. *J. Cancer Res. Clin. Oncol.* **2006**, *132*, 163–171. [CrossRef] [PubMed]
75. Plisiecka-Halasa, J. P21 WAF1, P27 KIP1 TP53 and C-MYC analysis in 204 ovarian carcinomas treated with platinum-based regimens. *Ann. Oncol.* **2003**, *14*, 1078–1085. [CrossRef] [PubMed]
76. Wu, C.C.; Hsu, Y.T.; Chang, C.L. Hyperthermicintraperitoneal chemotherapy enhances antitumor effects on ovarian cancer through immunemediated cancer stem cell targeting. *Int. J. Hyperth.* **2021**, *38*, 1013–1022. [CrossRef] [PubMed]
77. De Bree, E.; Katsougkri, D.; Polioudaki, H.; Tsangaridou, E.; Michelakis, D.; Zoras, O.; Theodoropoulos, P. Hyperthermia during Intraperitoneal Chemotherapy with Paclitaxel or Docetaxel for Ovarian Cancer: Is There Any Benefit? *Anticancer. Res.* **2020**, *40*, 6769–6780. [CrossRef]
78. Yarmolenko, P.S.; Moon, E.J.; Landon, C.; Manzoor, A.; Hochman, D.W.; Viglianti, B.L.; Dewhirst, M.W. Thresholds for thermal damage to normal tissues: An update. *Int. J. Hyperth.* **2011**, *27*, 320–343. [CrossRef]
79. Bear, A.S.; Kennedy, L.; Young, J.K.; Perna, S.K.; Almeida, J.P.M.; Lin, A.Y.; Eckels, P.C.; Drezek, R.A.; Foster, A.E. Elimination of metastatic melanoma using gold nanoshell-enabled photothermal therapy and adoptive T-cell transfer. *PLoS ONE* **2013**, *8*, e69073. [CrossRef]
80. Pelz, J.O.W.; Vetterlein, M.; Grimmig, T.; Kerscher, A.G.; Moll, E.; Lazariotou, M.; Matthes, N.; Faber, M.N.; Germer, C.-T.; Waaga-Gasser, A.M.; et al. Hyperthermic intraperitoneal chemotherapy in patients with peritoneal carcinomatosis: Role of heat-shock proteins and dissecting effects of hyperthermia. *Ann. Surg. Oncol.* **2013**, *20*, 1105–1113. [CrossRef]
81. Grimmig, T.; Moll, E.-M.; Kloos, K.; Thumm, R.; Moench, R.; Callies, S.; Kreckel, J.; Vetterlein, M.; Pelz, J.; Polat, B.; et al. Upregulated heat-shock proteins after hyperthermic chemotherapy point to induced cell survival mechanisms in affected tumor cells from peritoneal carcinomatosis. *Cancer Growth Metastasis* **2017**, *10*, 1179064417730559. [CrossRef]
82. Cesna, V.; Sukovas, A.; Jasukaitiene, A.; Silkuniene, G.; Paskauskas, S.; Dambrauskas, Z.; Gulbinas, A. Stimulated upregulation of HO-1 is associated with inadequate response of gastric and ovarian cancer cell lines to hyperthermia and cisplatin treatment. *Oncol. Lett.* **2019**, *18*, 1961–1968. [CrossRef]

Journal of
Clinical Medicine

MDPI

Article

Hyperthermic Intraperitoneal Chemotherapy and Recirculation with CO_2: A Safe Technique

Remedios Gómez-Sanz [1,2], Enrique Ovejero-Merino [1,2,*], Inmaculada Lasa-Unzúe [1], Adela López-García [1], Ruth Marcos-Hernández [1], Javier Mínguez-García [1], Francisca García-Moreno Nisa [1], Fernando Mendoza-Moreno [1], Manuel Díez-Alonso [1], Miguel A Ortega [3,4], Melchor Álvarez-Mon [3,4,5], Alberto Gutiérrez-Calvo [1,2] and the Spanish PRS Collaborating Group †

1 Department of General and Digestive Surgery, Príncipe de Asturias Teaching Hospital, 28805 Madrid, Spain
2 Spanish Group of Peritoneal Oncologic Surgery (GECOP), Principe de Asturias Teaching Hospital, University of Alcalá de Henares, 28001 Madrid, Spain
3 Department of Medicine and Medical Specialities, Faculty of Medicine and Health Sciences, University of Alcalá, 28801 Alcalá de Henares, Spain
4 Ramón y Cajal Institute of Sanitary Research (IRYCIS), Hospital Universitario Príncipe de Asturias, 28034 Madrid, Spain
5 Immune System Diseases-Rheumatology and Internal Medicine Service, University Hospital Príncipe de Asturias, (CIBEREHD), 28806 Alcalá de Henares, Spain
* Correspondence: enrique.ovejero@gmail.com; Tel.: +34-686-548-392
† Collaborators of the Spanish PRS Collaborating Group are indicated in the Supplementary Materials section.

Abstract: Introduction: Hyperthermic IntraPEritoneal Chemotherapy (HIPEC) has evolved as a treatment for peritoneal carcinomatosis in various tumors after a careful and complete cytoreductive surgery, and it demonstrated much better and longer survival than more traditional therapeutic schemas. Our objective has been to examine the safety, efficacy and survival achieved with closed technique with CO_2-agitation system Combat PRS® (Peritoneal Recirculation System: PRS). To achieve this, we compared the appearance of adverse events, mortality and survival with the described using classic techniques (open, closed without CO_2-agitation) for the treatment of selected patients with peritoneal carcinomatosis; Materials and methods: We studied overall survival, disease-free survival and safety (morbidity and mortality) of the administration of HIPEC through a closed method technique with CO_2 recirculation (Combat PRS®) in 482 patients from 11 Spanish hospitals; Results: The mortality of our technique (1.66%) was similar to other published techniques (open, closed). Morbidity exhibited a 9.96% rate of Clavien-Dindo (CD) III/IV complications in 482 patients, which was lower than in other series. Survival (overall survival (OS) and disease-free survival (DFS)) was similar to previously published results: 86% 1y-OS, 54% 3y-OS, 77% 1y-DFS and 31% 3y-DFS; Conclusion: The procedure with closed PRS with CO_2 agitation is as safe as standard open and closed procedures for the administration of HIPEC after complete cytoreductive surgery, with similar and very low mortality (1.66%) and lower morbidity (9.96% CD III and IV in our series vs range of 20–40% in the majority of different series); only Kusamura had similar results, with 12% in 205 patients, using the closed technique without CO_2 agitation).

Keywords: peritoneal carcinomatosis; intraperitoneal chemotherapy; cytoreductive surgery; intraoperative intraperitoneal chemotherapy; Spanish PRS Group

1. Introduction

The combination of cytoreductive surgery and perioperative chemotherapy [1–7] is the treatment of choice for select patients with peritoneal carcinomatosis of many tumors (e.g., peritoneal pseudomyxoma, mesothelioma or colon tumors [8–10]), and it has great promise in other tumor types [11] (e.g., gastric [12–15] or ovarian origin [1,2,16]).

Cytoreductive surgery (CRS) aims to completely remove all macroscopically visible tumors, and perioperative chemotherapy (CT) acts in a complementarily way to eradicate microscopic residual implants [4–6]. Although cytoreductive surgery procedures have become quite standardized since the publication of peritonectomy techniques by Sugarbaker, this standardization has not occurred with intraperitoneal chemotherapy, which has many existing protocols involving different chemotherapeutic drugs, durations, temperatures and application methods. [17].

CRS with intraoperative chemotherapy are usually long and complex procedures, usually involving multivisceral and peritoneal resections, with great systemic surgical repercussion and the added toxicity of concomitant, intraoperative and chemotherapy, but the long-term results are encouraging [4,18,19].

The HIPEC rationale is deliver a higher dosage of chemotherapy on the locoregional extension of the tumor (the peritoneal surface) with lower systemic toxicity. The direct introduction of chemotherapy in the peritoneal cavity achieves this objective, but this is further improved by hyperthermia, which enhances the penetration depth of cytotoxic drugs. This depth is limited and, therefore, can be only effective in patients with minimal residual disease after complete CRS [20].

The drugs, methods of application and timing of chemotherapy, however differ between work groups, and new techniques and methods have evolved to optimize the application of chemotherapeutic agents. Although HIPEC is the most widely used procedure in leading oncological centers, it lacks uniformity [2,6,21], with extensive variability in chemotherapeutic drugs, chemotherapeutic contact durations and methods of administration. Open, closed, half-open techniques or treatment with peritoneal cavity expansion coexist with the most recent contributions of a laparoscopic method (PIPAC) and closed technique with CO_2 agitation (Combat PRS®). The best technique remains controversial [22].

Theoretical advantages of a closed system with CO_2 agitation (Combat PRS®) are to maintain a more constant temperature within the peritoneal cavity, to achieve a homogeneous distribution of the chemotherapy selected and diminish the risk for operating system, as its assembly is easy and staff have minimal contact with chemotherapy (only during final aspiration of the abdominal cavity); this has been tested in pigs [23]).

Our objective is to examine whether the closed technique with the CO_2-agitation system (Combat PRS®) was a safe and effective treatment of select patients with peritoneal carcinomatosis in real world practice, in 11 hospitals in Spain.

2. Materials and Methods

This study was a multi-center, retrospective study of 11 Spanish hospitals (Table 1, Figure 1a–d) that used the closed technique with CO_2 agitation (Combat PRS®, Madrid, Spain) in the context of the multidisciplinary treatment of peritoneal carcinomatosis.

Table 1. Participating hospitals, patients provided (yearly tumoral histology) and evolution over time of the number of procedures. (Pseud: pseudomyxoma. Perit: primary peritoneal. Mesot: peritoneal mesothelioma. Sarco: peritoneal sarcoma. Append: appendix. Panc: pancreas).

Series	Colon	Ovarian	Gastric	Pseud.	Perit.	Mesot.	Sarco.	Append.	Panc.	Other	Total
2011		3									3
2012		10									10
2013	5	14	1								20
2014	15	8	9			2		1			35
2015	28	14	10	2		1	1	4			60
2016	28	25	9	4		1		3		1	71
2017	55	20	8	11	1	2		5	1	1	104
2018	70	46	11	14	1	2	1		6	2	153
2019	9	9	1	1		2		1	2	1	26

Table 1. *Cont.*

Series	Colon	Ovarian	Gastric	Pseud.	Perit.	Mesot.	Sarco.	Append.	Panc.	Other	Total
Total	210	149	49	32	2	10	2	14	9	5	482

	Cumulative Series 2019
Fuenlabrada University Hospital	101
Cuidad Real University Hospital	79
Principe de Asturias University Hospital	85
Gran Canaria Insular Hospital	71
Madrid Sanchinarro University Hospital	47
University of Malaga Regional University Hospital	45
Fundación Alcorcon University Hospital	18
Elche General University Hospital	14
Reina Sofia University Hospital	14
FJD University Hospital	2
Virgen de Arraixaca University Hospital	6
TOTAL	482

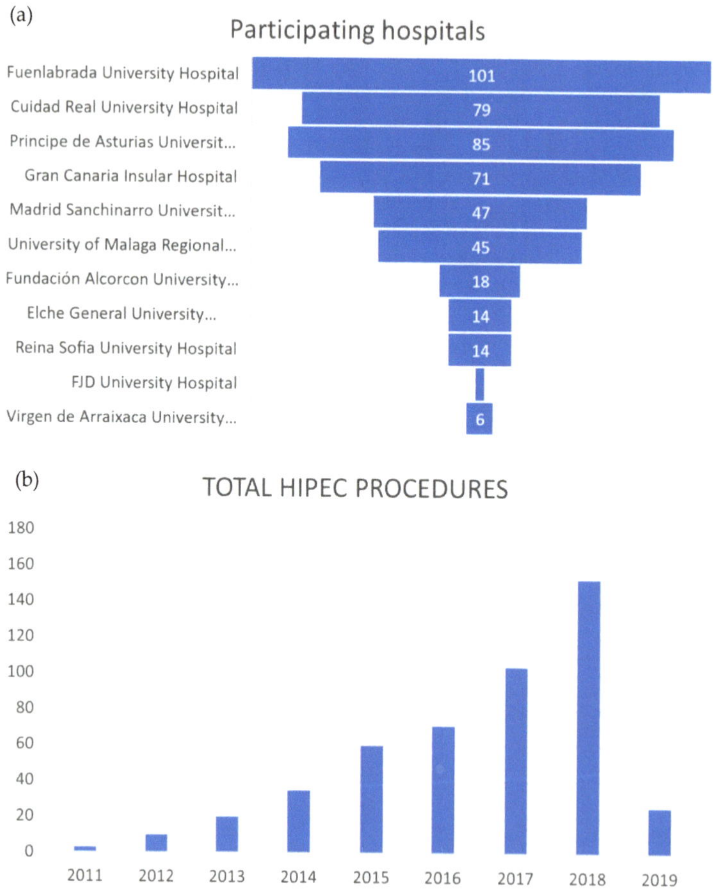

Figure 1. *Cont.*

(c)

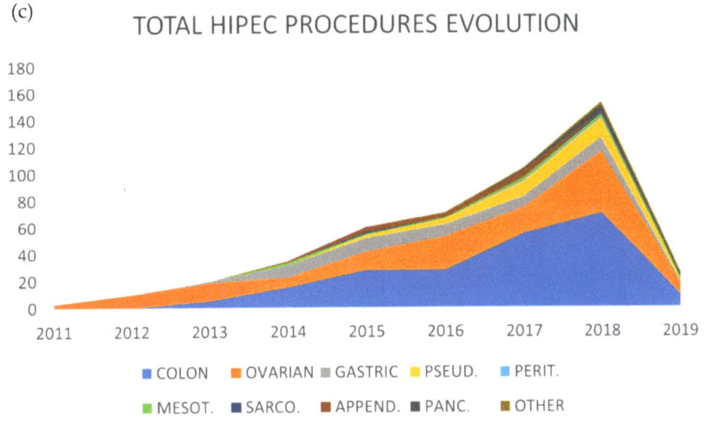

(d)

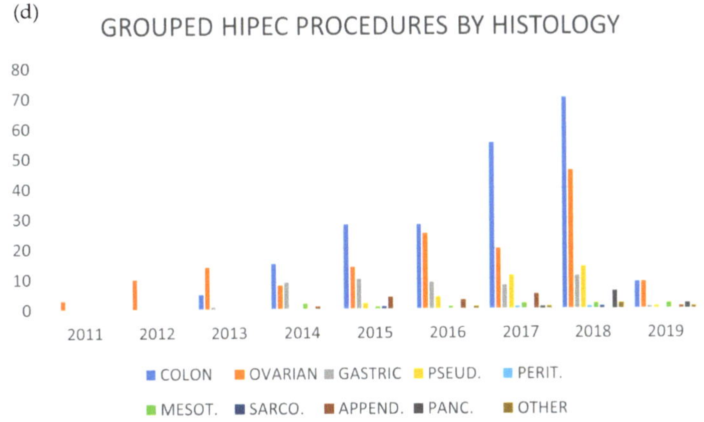

Figure 1. (**a**) Eleven participating hospitals. (**b**) Yearly increase of total HIPEC procedures. (**c**) Yearly increase of HIPEC procedures, with area proportional to histology, showing than the two main histologies are colon and ovarian origin. (**d**) Yearly evolution of HIPEC procedures with disaggregated yearly histology.

The study period was from 2011 to February 2019, with a gradual and strong increase in the number of patients treated using this technique during this period (Table 2, Figure 2a,b).

Table 2. Types of tumours.

Tumour	Total	%	Clinical PCI	Surgery PCI
Colon	210	43.6	4.6 (3.89–5.31)	6.37 (5.44–7.30)
Ovarian	149	30.9	8.58 (7.47–9.70)	9.68 (8.49–10.88)
Gastric	49	10.2	4.04 (2.12–5.96)	4.89 (2.81–6.98)
Appendix	14	2.9	8.64 (7.54–9.30)	10.33 (9.25–11.10)
Pseudomixoma	32	6.6	8.59 (7.20–9.70)	11.78 (10.50–12.36)
Mesothelioma	10	2.1	19.63 (17.25–20.50)	21.78 (18.30–22.45)
Pancreas	9	1.9		
Other	4	0.8		
Primary peritoneal	2	0.4		
Endometrium	1	0.2		
Sarcoma	2	0.4		
Total	482	100%		

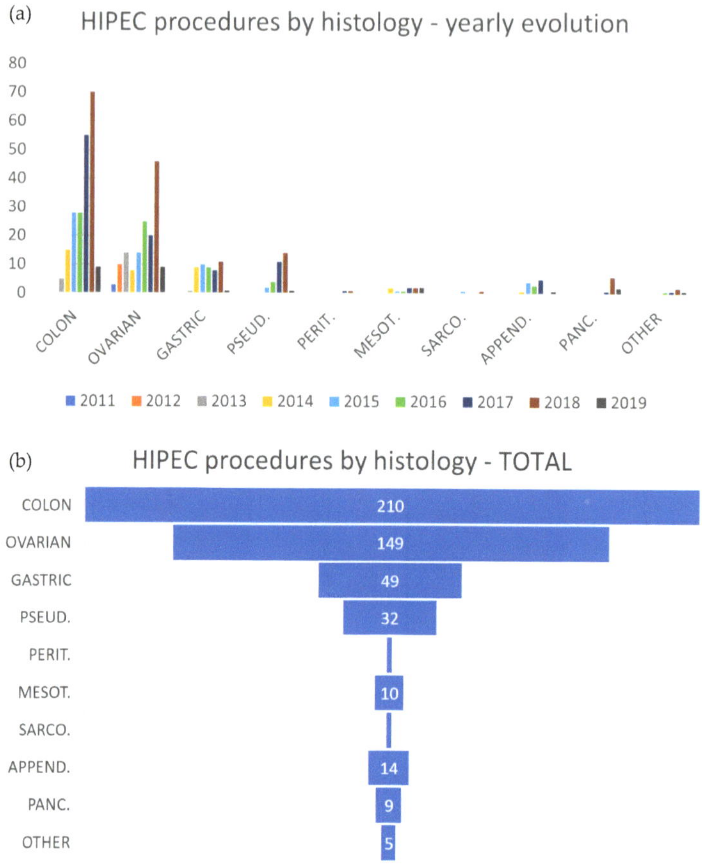

Figure 2. (**a**) Histology: yearly evolution of HIPEC procedures. (**b**) Total HIPEC procedures by histology.

The study included 482 patients who met the specific inclusion criteria (Table 3). All patients received HIPEC with a CO_2-agitation system and the same perfusion machine (Combat PRS®). The surgical approach in every case was the one described by Sugarbaker [17]. The chemotherapeutics used and the treatment time varied according to the preferred protocol of each participating center.

Table 3. Inclusion criteria [24].

- Complete Cytoreduction (R0 resective surgery)
- Age < 75 years
- Functional Status According to WHO (ECOG) ≤ 2
- Presence of Peritoneal Carcinomatosis
- Absence of Extra-Abdominal Metastasis
- Absence of Hepatic Metastasis requiring a major or nonresectable hepatectomy
- Liver, Kidney and Bone Marrow function within these parameters:
    - Total Bilirubin $\leq$ 1.5 times the upper limit of normal (ULN)
    - GOT/GPT $\leq$ 2.5 times ULN
    - AP $\leq$ 3 times ULN
    - Serum Creatinine $\leq$ 1.5 times NFS
    - Neutrophils > 1.5 × 103
    - Hb > 10 g/dL
    - Platelets > 100,000

Twenty-four variables were collected in a prospective database created for this purpose. The carcinomatosis index was quantified according to the peritoneal cancer index (PCI) described by Sugarbaker [25–27]. Data were collected on intraoperative complications related to the surgery, and data linked to HIPEC were collected separately. Complications detected in the postoperative period were recorded and codified according to the 2004 version of the Clavien-Dindo (CD) scale [28]. (Clavien-Dindo I and II are deviations from normal postoperative course solved pharmacologically; CD III are complications which require surgical/endoscopic or radiologic intervention without (IIIa) or with (IIIb) general anesthesia, and CD IV are life-threatening complications that require admission to Intensive Care Unit (ICU), with single organ (IVa) or multiorgan (IVb) disfunction. CD V is death: "mortality"). For the analysis of morbidity, CD III and IV have been taken into account (as reported in the main articles of Table 4).

Table 4. Comparison of morbidity/mortality and survival among various series related to the HIPEC technique used.

Authors	Technique	No.	Year	Tumour	Mortality (%)	Morbidity (%)	OS	DFS	Classification
Sugarbaker et al. [29]	Open	356	2006	AP	2	19	-	-	IV (proprietary base)
Elias et al. [30]	Open Closed	523	2010	CRC	3.3	31	1 y: 81% 3 y: 41% 5 y: 27%	1 y: 47% 3 y: 15% 5 y: 10%	CD: III/IV CTCAE
Goére [11] (PSOGI)	Open Closed	781	2017	Rare OC, Sarcomas, NT	2.9	41	1 y: 78% 3 y: 52% 5 y: 39%	1 y: 61% 3 y: 33% 5 y: 28%	CTCAE 4
Glehen et al. [31]	Closed	207	2003	OC, CRC, GC, PMP, PM, others	3.2	24.5	-	-	CD: III/IV
Kusamura et al. [32]	Closed	205	2006	OC, CRC, GC, PMP, PM, others	0.9	12	-	-	Bozzetti: 3–4
Levine et al. [33]	Closed	460	2007	OC, CRC, GC, PMP, PM, PS, others	4.8	43	3 y: 60%	-	Not described
Manzanedo et al. [15] (GECOP)	Open Closed PRS	88	2019	GC	3.4	31	1 y: 80% 3 y: 31%	1 y: 46% 3 y: 22%	CD (v2004): III/IV
Sanchez-Garcia et al. [34]	Closed PRS	21	2016	OC	4.76	38.1	-	-	CD: III/IV CTCAE 4
Cianci [35]	Closed PRS	17	2018	CRC, OC, AP, GC	0	38.1	-	-	CD: III/IV
Our group (Spain)	Closed PRS	482	2019	CRC, AP, GC, PMP, OC, others	1.66	9.96	1 y: 86% 3 y: 54%	1 y: 77% 3 y: 31%	CD (v2004): III/IV

GC: gastric cancer. CRC: colorectal cancer. AP: appendiceal cancer. OC: ovarian cancer. PMP: pseudomyxoma. PM: peritoneal mesothelioma. NT: neuroendocrine tumor. CTCAE: Common Terminology Criteria for Adverse Events. CD: Clavien-Dindo. GECOP: Spanish group of peritoneal oncologic surgery. Note: "Mortality" equals Clavien-Dindo V. 1 y: 1 year. 3 y: 3 year. 5 y: 5 year.

IBM-SPSS, version 22 (IBM, Armonk, NY, USA), was used for statistical analyses. Actual survival was calculated using Kaplan–Meier curves.

Description of HIPEC Administration Technique

The closed technique with CO_2 agitation is based on the existence of two closed circuits. One circuit is filled with chemotherapy agents, and the other circuit is filled with gas bubbles (CO_2).

After complete cytoreduction and exposure of all appropriate abdominal cavities, the base of the control device was passed through a small orifice (2 cm) in the abdominal wall to connect the cavity to a transparent extracorporeal cylinder (Figure 3a,b) that allowed us to monitor the proper level of filling and the intraabdominal pressure (which was approximately equal to the height of the water column over the skin level within this control device). This device was held in a vertical and stable position by an external arm tightly attached to the operating table. The three thinner multiperforated tubes for gas intake (Figure 3a (light green)) were positioned under the intestinal package and extended like a trident at the root of the mesentery. All tubes converged into a single tube, which exited the cavity through another small (1 cm) skin orifice over the left iliac fossa. This tube may be used to place a drain at the end of the procedure. A recirculation circuit of CO_2 was established between these tubes (gas inlet) and the upper part of the control device (gas outlet (Figure 3a (black dot)).

Chemotherapeutic drugs in a liquid carrier solution were administered (inflow) via specially designed, multiperforated Y-shaped tubes with blunt ends (Figure 3a (white)), which were exteriorized through the lower part of the laparotomy and placed superficially over the visceral package. After entering the abdominal cavity, the solution was recovered (outflow) and recirculated through similar tubes with a larger diameter than the gas tubes (Figure 3a (blue)), which were exteriorized through the upper end of the laparotomy and positioned deeply in both parietocolic gutters. Once the tubes were placed, the laparotomy was closed as tightly as possible using continuous blocking stitches in the skin to allow impregnation of the abdominal wall with the chemotherapeutic agents during recirculation. After skin closure, recirculation of the solvent/carrier solution (transport liquid without chemotherapy) was started to test patency without external contamination risk. The solvent was generally the same liquid used for peritoneal dialysis (Physioneal 35, with 1.36% glucose) and preheated to 42 °C. After verification of correct recirculation, the gas was introduced to test the gas circuit. Once the desired amount of CO_2 had been introduced, it only recirculated within its own circuit. Chemotherapeutic agents were added after confirmation that both circuits were functioning properly. Recirculation of CO_2 aims to cause a turbulent flow that ensures a homogenous mixture of the chemotherapeutic agent solution and heat throughout the entire abdominal cavity.

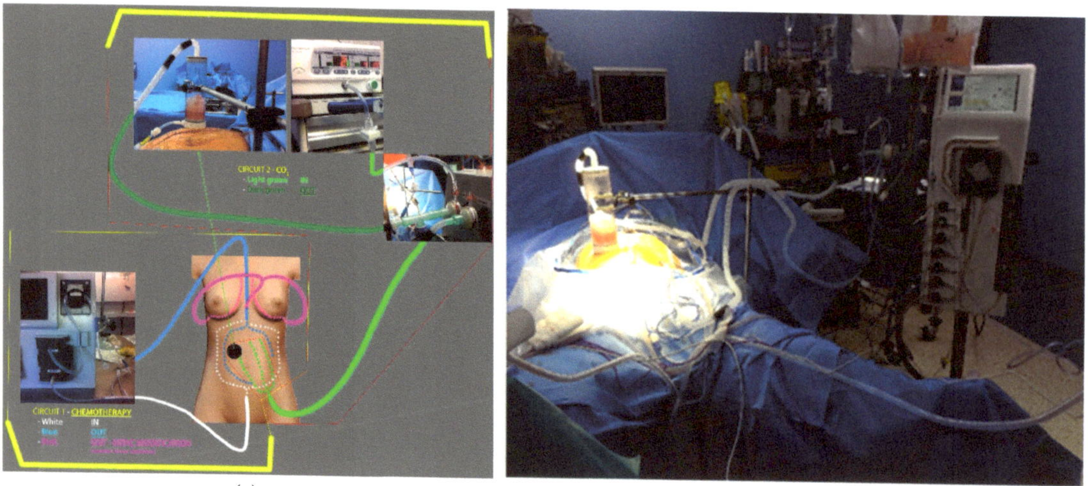

(a) (b)

Figure 3. HIPEC and HITAC schematic view. Part (**a**) schematic view of the HIPEC system (white IN-blue OUT for chemotherapy, light green IN-dark green OUT for CO_2; in pink, the HITAC modification, allowing chemotherapy recover from pleural cavities. Part (**b**) real intraoperative setting of HIPEC with Combat PRS®(Author: E. Ovejero-Merino).

The dose of chemotherapy was calculated according to the surface area of the patient's body, and the amount of transport fluid depended on the capacity of each patient's abdominal cavity, tissue compliance and degree of anaesthetic relaxation.

After completion of the recirculation time, the cavity was drained via the outlet tubes. Two full 5-min washes were performed with a clean, gas-free recirculation liquid to remove any remnant chemotherapeutic agents. After the last wash, the abdominal cavity was reopened, and any remaining liquid was manually suctioned. All disposable material was removed from the patient and directly placed into biological waste buckets to minimize the risk of contamination of operating room staff.

The diagram presents the variation used when it was necessary to open or resect any part of the diaphragm, which allowed cells to potentially reach the pleural cavity. This variation allowed perfusion and recovery of the recirculation fluid from the pleural cavity during the perfusion by connecting chest tubes to the outlet tubes. This variation was named HIperthermic ThoracoAbdominal Chemotherapy (HITAC).

3. Results

3.1. Description of the Series

Of the 482 patients, 66.4% were women and 33.6% were men. The average age at the time of the surgery was 59 years (CI $\pm$ 11.39).

In total, 210 cases were colon tumors, 149 cases were ovarian tumors, 49 cases were gastric tumors, 32 cases were pseudomyxoma, 14 cases were appendiceal tumors, 10 cases were mesothelioma, 2 cases were primary peritoneal tumors and 16 cases were other tumors (i.e., 9 pancreas, 1 endometrial, 2 sarcomas, 1 neuroendocrine and 3 GIST) (Table 2).

The global mean hospital stay was 13.4 days with 3.2 days in the ICU. There were no significant differences related to the type of tumor.

For the procedures performed in the cytoreduction, more than four procedures were performed in 215 patients (44.6%).

3.2. Peritoneal Carcinomatosis Index (PCI)

The clinical PCI was lower than the PCI during surgery in all the included tumors (Table 2).

3.3. Chemotherapeutic Drugs

For colon tumors, the most commonly used agents were mitomycin C for 60 to 90 min (46.2%) and oxaliplatin for 30 min (45.7%).

The preferred drugs for ovarian tumors were paclitaxel (61.7%) and the combination cisplatin/doxorubicin (16.1%) for 60 min.

For gastric carcinomatosis, the most frequent combination (42.9%) was cisplatin and mitomycin C for 60 min.

For pseudomyxoma tumors, mitomycin C for 60 min was used in 78.1% of the cases.

For mesothelioma tumors, most cases (66.6%) received the combination cisplatin and doxorubicin for 90 min.

3.4. Morbidity/Mortality

A total of 170 patients (35.27%) exhibited complications during their hospital stay, and we classified the adverse events using the Clavien-Dindo scale. Only 48 of these adverse events (9.96%) were serious (CD III/IV) (Table 5).

Table 5. Part **(a)** Relation between variables and increased morbidity; Part **(b)** Postoperative deaths (Clavien-Dindo V) (Decade 1 = 0–9 years; decade 2 = 10–19 years, and so on); Part **(c)** HIPEC specifically-related complications (CD II).

(a)

Complications CD III/IV	Statistic	p Value	Risk	CI
>4 procedures	Chi squared	0.035	1.928	(1.16–3.20)
Surgical PCI	Mann–Whitney U	0.154		
Age	Mann–Whitney U	0.888		
Type of primary tumour	Chi squared	0.387		
Medicine	Chi squared	0.103		
Sex	Chi squared	0.088		
HIPEC time	Mann–Whitney U	0.793		

(b)

Case ID	Age (Decade)	Histology	Postop Day	HIPEC Drugs	HIPEC Time	ICU Days	Cause of Death
HUCR11	7 th	Ovarian	8	Paclitaxel	60	7	Probable PE, CRA
HUCR35	8 th	Ovarian	12	Paclitaxel	60	8	Intestinal perforation Peritonitis Multi-organ failure
HUCR36	7 th	Ovarian	3	Paclitaxel	60	17	Intestinal perforation Intestinal ischemia Multi-organ failure
HMS12	5 th	Colon	17	Oxaliplatin	60	79	Sepsis
HMS34	8 th	Colon	20	Oxaliplatin	45	18	MI
HUPA70	6 th	Pseudomyxoma	35	Mitomycin C + 5FU + Folinic	90	3	PE
HRUM18	8 th	Colon	3	Oxaliplatin	30	8	Post-operative LGIB
HUFLB	10 th	Colon		Oxaliplatin	30	8	Fatal and unexpected liver failure

(c)

Code	Age (Decade)	T. 1°	>4 Proc	PCI PRE-SURGICAL	PCI IN SURGERY	HIPEC Drugs	Time	Complication	Days in ICU
HUPA34	8 th	Colon	Yes	7	6	Oxaliplatin + Leucovorin + 5FU	10	Anaphylactic shock	7
HRUM12	4 th	Colon	Yes	30	30	Oxaliplatin	30	Hyperglycaemia	2
HRUM15	7 th	Colon	No	4	4	Oxaliplatin	30	Metabolic acidosis	2
HRUM18	7 th	Colon	No	3	3	Oxaliplatin	30	Hyperglycaemia	8
HRUM21	5 th	Ovary	No	2	3	Cisplatin + Doxorrubicin	90	Hyperglycaemia	2
HRUM22	7 th	Colon	No	6	23	Oxaliplatin	30	Hyperglycaemia	2
HRUM30	6 th	Colon	Yes	4	7	Mitomycin	60	Hyperglycaemia	2
HRUM40	6 th	Colon	No	2	3	Oxaliplatin	30	Hyperglycaemia	3
HGUE	5 th	Ovary	Yes	13	13	Paclitaxel	45	Hypercarbia	3

PE: pulmonary embolism. CRA: cardiorespiratory arrest. MI: acute myocardial infarction. LGIB: lower gastrointestinal bleeding.

Variables, such as age, drug used, PCI, type of primary tumor or HIPEC time, were not associated with increased morbidity. Only the number of procedures > 4 was significantly linked to an increase in morbidity.

Eight patients died in the postoperative period (1.66%). Four deaths were due to medical causes (PE, MI and liver failure), and the other deaths were due to causes directly related to the surgery (intestinal perforation, sepsis and lower GI bleeding). None of these deaths were directly related to the administration of HIPEC.

We found nine cases with complications that were linked exclusively to HIPEC (detected during the procedure) (1.9% of the total): six hyperglycaemia cases over 400 mg/dL, one allergy to oxaliplatin (anaphylactic shock), one significant metabolic acidosis and one case of hypercarbia (the only directly relatable with CO_2 agitation). Seven cases were colon carcinomatosis (two appendiceal), and two cases were ovarian. The HIPEC duration was

30 min in 5 of the nine cases. The complications linked to HIPEC did not significantly increase the stay in the ICU.

Hyperglycaemia >400 mg/dL was related to carrier solution (5% dextrose) and was avoided, and in further procedures, carrier solution was switched to peritoneal dialysis fluid (Physioneal 35, with 1.36% glucose). With no known clinical significance of the difference, 5% dextrose maintains a concentration of oxaliplatin at levels that reach 101.2% at 60′ and 105.1% at 120′ of HIPEC, while peritoneal dialysis fluid levels slowly decrease to 91.7% at 60′ and 85.3% at 120′ of the original dosage, but avoids the serious hyperglycaemia and electrolyte disturbances caused by the former (5% dextrose). [36].

3.5. Survival Curves

The OS of the series with a mean follow-up of 17.8 months was 86.1% and 54.1% after the first and third years, with DFS rates of 77.2% and 31.4%, respectively; a direct comparison with the main series can be seen in Tables 4 and 6 and Figure 4. The data by tumoral histology are detailed in Figure 2.

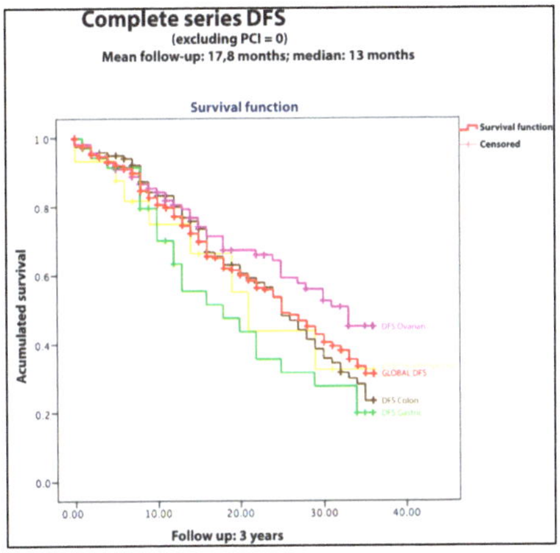

(a)

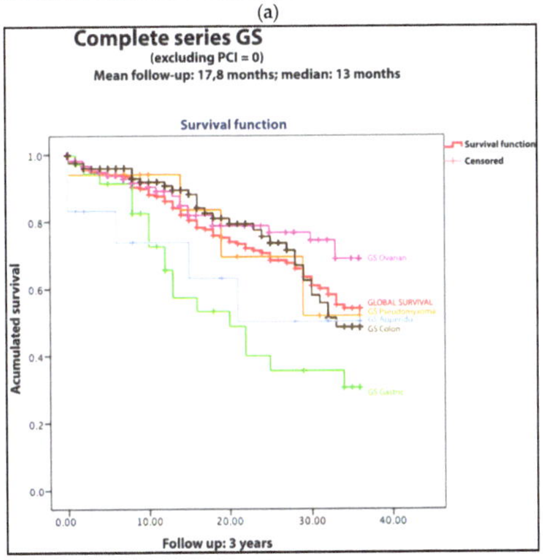

(b)

Figure 4. Survival curves by histology. (**a**) DFS: disease-free survival; ovarian (pink), global group (red), pseudomyxoma (orange) appendix (blue), colon (brown), gastric (green). (**b**) GS: global survival); ovarian (pink), pseudomyxoma (yellow), global group (red), colon (brown), gastric (green).

Table 6. OS and DFS, by tumour histology, 1 and 3 years after HIPEC procedure.

Tumour Origin	Mean Follow-Up (Months)	OS 1 Year	OS 3 Years	DFS 1 Year	DFS 3 Years
Colon carcinomatosis	17.7	90.7%	48.7%	80.1%	23.4%
Appendiceal carcinomatosis	17.5	92.3%	64.6%	75.2%	51.6%
Ovarian carcinomatosis	18.8	89.1%	68.9%	80.8%	45.2%
Gastric carcinomatosis	17.3	65.8%	30.6%	63.5%	19.8%
Pseudomyxoma	14	84.2%	52.6%	76.3%	33.9%
Mesothelioma	16.2	50%	50%	50%	30%

4. Discussion

Cytoreductive surgery in the treatment of peritoneal carcinomatosis is a useful tool in centers with experience and appropriate patient selection [37] to increase overall and disease-free survival [38,39]. The rate of complications in these procedures, which sometimes require excision of the peritoneum and the resection of affected organs for the macroscopic elimination of the tumor, is very similar to other highly complex surgeries [38].

The role of intraperitoneal chemotherapy as a theoretical complementary treatment to surgery for the eradication of the residual microscopic tumor has not been completely demonstrated in prospective trials [40,41], which may be because it has a much less standardized protocol than surgery [42]. Therefore, each group uses different treatment protocols with different chemotherapeutic agents, times, temperatures and methods of application without any evidence of which protocol produces better results [39,43]. Therefore, it is difficult to obtain global and valid conclusions. Intraperitoneal chemotherapy is also used in other scenarios, such as the prophylaxis treatment of peritoneal carcinomatosis in high-risk tumors [44] or the treatment of malignant ascites [45].

Intraperitoneal chemotherapy acts directly on local tumor cells via various mechanisms. The chemotherapeutic drugs selected are generally hydrophiles, with high molecular-weight molecules to prevent the drugs from passing through the peritoneal barrier. This characteristic minimizes their passage into the bloodstream, decreases their systemic toxicity and achieves much higher intraperitoneal concentrations than would be possible or safe with systemic chemotherapy [46]. The selected agents must have a fast, direct cytotoxic effect on the residual tumor, which must not be larger than 2.5 mm because the chemotherapeutic agents will not completely permeate the full thickness of larger tumors during the recirculation time.

Hyperthermia theoretically acts in three ways [47–51]: the first mechanism produces a direct thermal cytotoxic effect on the tumor cell; the second mechanism increases the cytotoxicity of the chemotherapeutic agents; and the third mechanism increases the ability of the chemotherapeutic agent to penetrate inside tumoral implants. Hyperthermia itself seems to play a significant role in the efficacy of intraperitoneal chemotherapy, as Yonemura et al. founded: "HIPEC at 42–43 °C had better results than lower temperatures or no HIPEC (only CRS)" [52], but the ideal temperature in a varied range of chemotherapeutic agents still remains controversial, because not all chemotherapeutic drugs reach their maximum efficacy or stability at the same temperature [49]. Some recent publications related high temperatures (>41.4 °C) to lower survival rates [14], and other studies related these findings to the synthesis of heat shock proteins (HSP) inside tumor cells, which ultimately protected the tumor cells ("thermotolerance") by reducing the apoptosis generated by the chemotherapeutic drugs or selecting the subpopulations of tumor cells that were most resistant to the administered chemotherapy [50]. HSP therapies are being investigated to prevent their protective actions and as a marker for cytotoxic drugs [47].

Therefore, the ideal temperature is not well defined and will likely vary depending on the drugs used when we have more knowledge of their behavior at high temperatures. However, we must be able to monitor the temperature of the chemotherapy very well, modify it and keep it constant and homogeneous within the cavity for maximum efficacy in all areas and to avoid heat damage in areas of possible accumulation.

Another significant influence on the efficacy of intraperitoneal chemotherapy is the intraabdominal pressure of the fluid. Increasing the intraabdominal pressure increases the penetration of the medicine into the cell layers of the tumor implant by collapsing the capillaries that wash the chemotherapeutic agents in the peritoneum and increases the concentration and permanence of the agent in contact with the tumoral cells [45,53].

The most widely used method for the administration of perioperative chemotherapy is Hyperthermic IntraPEritoneal Chemotherapy (HIPEC) [22,54] because it unites the cytotoxic effect of chemotherapeutic agents with the effect of thermal shock on tumor cells. The classic method described by P. Sugarbaker is the open or "Coliseum" method, in which the chemotherapeutic agents are dissolved in a carrier solution, enter the abdominal cavity and are manually moved continuously to reach all areas of the peritoneum. However, the great difficulty of this method is maintaining a constant temperature throughout the entire abdomen. There are also safety concerns because of the direct and long-term contact of the surgeons with the chemotherapeutic drugs. A closed method was subsequently described to avoid possible exposure of the staff to the chemotherapeutic agents and maintain a more homogeneous temperature within the cavity and a higher intraabdominal pressure to help the penetration of chemotherapeutic agents into the tumor cells. The problem with this technique is the early formation of adhesions that hinder the ability to reach all areas of the peritoneum and the potential accumulation of heat or chemotherapeutic agents in some areas, which could lead to lesions or increased toxicity [22].

After several experimental trials in pigs [23] verified the safety of the technique, we started to use a new method for the administration of HIPEC in 2012, which was the closed technique with CO_2 recirculation (Combat PRS®, Madrid, Spain).

Regarding efficacy, our results are very promising, with a mean overall survival near 50% at 3 years in a pathology where the published survival without treatment is 6 months (49% in colon cancer, almost 70% in ovarian cancer and 30% for tumors when carcinomatosis appears as gastric cancer).

The grade III/IV morbidity of our series was 9.96%, which is within the expected range for a surgery of this complexity and consistent with other groups. The mortality was also within acceptable margins and was 1.66% in our series [40].

Various studies compared the classic open and closed methods, but no groups demonstrated that one procedure was better than the other. Therefore, the best application method of HIPEC remains controversial [1,2].

In our experience, morbidity was lower by using the closed technique with CO_2 in comparison with previous literature [1–9]; thus, it seems to be a safe option. As the different studies used different systems to classify adverse events, a direct comparison using a metanalysis review is unfortunately not possible [28].

Based on the morbidity/mortality data of the entire process and the analysis of the complications directly related to HIPEC, we found that the severe adverse events were related either to the chemotherapeutic drug itself (anaphylactic shock) or the carrier medium (hyperglycemia). Only one case presented a plausibly related complication with CO_2 agitaton, hypercarbia, and survived.

During the procedures, no accidents were documented for spillage or contamination of the operating room staff with the chemotherapeutic agents. One advantage for the Combat PRS® system is it is easy to mount and the cavity is closed and the gas is recirculated through the device, and thus the risk of inhaling any vapor created when heating the medicine is reduced to a minimum. Therefore, the procedure is also safe for health care staff when it is performed in compliance with the established protocol and security measures.

A main limitation of the study is the variability between centers because each center used a different treatment regimen with different chemotherapeutic drugs and times. These differences make it difficult for a comparison of concrete chemotherapy added or time of the technique. The variability in protocol as well as different length of follow-up in the included patients will require additional studies.

5. Conclusions

According to the experience of our multi-center group, the closed system with CO_2 agitation seems to be a safe procedure for the application of HIPEC for the patient and health care staff. Only one patient suffered hypercarbia, which could be related directly to the CO_2 agitation use. This new protocol showed similar survival as the previously published series. The application of HIPEC with CO_2 recirculation using the Combat PRS® device, thus, seems to be a safe and effective procedure that may be added to the therapeutic arsenal in the multimodal treatment of peritoneal carcinomatosis.

Supplementary Materials: The following supporting information can be downloaded at: https://www.mdpi.com/article/10.3390/jcm11206152/s1, Spanish PRS collaborating group: Dr. Israel Manzanedo, on behalf of the Department of General and Digestive Surgery, Hospital Universitario Fuenlabrada, Madrid, Spain. Dra. Susana Sánchez García, on behalf of the Department of General and Digestive Surgery, Hospital Universitario of Ciudad Real. Dra. Laura González Sánchez, on behalf of the Department of General and Digestive Surgery Hospital Insular de Gran Canaria. Dr. Eduardo Díaz Reques, on behalf of the Department of General and Digestive Surgery, Hospital Universitario Madrid Sanchinarro. Dr. Alberto Titos García, on behalf of the Department of General and Digestive Surgery, Hospital Regional Universitario de Málaga. Dr. Manuel E. Marcello Fernández, on behalf of Hospital Universitario Fundación Alcorcón, Madrid, Spain. Dr. Ibán Caravaca García, on behalf of Hospital General Universitario de Elche, Alicante, Spain. Dr. Álvaro Arjona, on behalf of the Department of General and Digestive Surgery, Hospital Reina Sofía, Córdoba, Spain. Dr. Pedro Villarejo Campos, on behalf of Hospital Universitario Fundación Jiménez Díaz. Dr. Pedro Cascales Campos, on behalf of the Department of General and Digestive Surgery, Hospital Virgen de la Arrixaca, Murcia, Spain.

Author Contributions: Conceptualization, R.G.-S. and E.O.-M., investigation, R.G.-S., E.O.-M., I.L.-U., A.L.-G., R.M.-H., J.M.-G., F.G.-M.N., F.M.-M., M.D.-A., M.A.O., M.Á.-M. and A.G.-C.; writing—original draft preparation, R.G.-S., E.O.-M., I.L.-U., A.L.-G., R.M.-H., J.M.-G., F.G.-M.N., F.M.-M., M.D.-A. and A.G.-C.; writing—review and editing, R.G.-S., E.O.-M., I.L.-U., A.L.-G., R.M.-H., J.M.-G., F.G.-M.N., F.M.-M., M.D.-A., M.A.O., M.Á.-M. and A.G.-C.; supervision; R.G.-S. and E.O.-M., project administration, M.A.O.; funding acquisition, M.Á.-M. and M.A.O. All authors have read and agreed to the published version of the manuscript.

Funding: This study was supported by the Instituto de Salud Carlos III (Plan Estatal de I + D + I 2013–2016) and co-financed by the European Development Regional Fund "A way to achieve Europe" (ERDF) and B2017/BMD-3804 MITIC-CM, B2020/MITICAD-CM, HALEKULANY and MJR.

Institutional Review Board Statement: The study was carried out in accordance with the basic ethical principles of autonomy, beneficence, nonmaleficence and distributive justice, and its development followed the rules of Good Clinical Practice, the principles contained in the most recent Declaration of Helsinki (2013) and the Oviedo Convention (1997). The collected data and information complied with the current legislation on data protection (Organic Law 3/5 December 2018 on the Protection of Personal Data and the Guarantee of Digital Rights and Regulation (EU) 2016/679) approved by Hospital Universitario Principe de Asturias (0E17/2019).

Informed Consent Statement: Informed consent was obtained from all subjects involved in the study.

Data Availability Statement: The data used to support the findings of the present study are available from the corresponding author upon request.

Conflicts of Interest: The authors declare no conflict of interest. Founding Role supported by COMBAT®. Role of the Funding Source: initial study of device regulatory approvals and external biostatistics analysis; the funders had no role in the design of the study; in the collection, or interpretation of data; in the writing of the manuscript; or in the decision to publish the results.

References

1. Roviello, F.; Caruso, S.; Marrelli, D.; Pedrazzani, C.; Neri, A.; De Stefano, A.; Pinto, E. Treatment of peritoneal carcinomatosis with cytoreductive surgery and hyperthermic intraperitoneal chemotherapy: State of the art and future developments. *Surg. Oncol.* **2011**, *20*, e38–e54. [CrossRef] [PubMed]
2. Glehen, O.; Mohamed, F.; Gilly, F.N. Peritoneal carcinomatosis from digestive tract cancer: New management by cytoreductive surgery and intraperitoneal chemohyperthermia. *Lancet Oncol.* **2004**, *5*, 219–228. [CrossRef]
3. Gómez-Portilla, A.; Cendoya, I.; de Tejada, I.L.; Olabarriaa, I.; Magrach, L.; de Lecea, C.M.; Gil, A.; Valdovinos, M.; Larrabide, I.; de Alegría, N.R. Bases y fundamentos del tratamiento de la carcinomatosis peritoneal por cáncer colorrectal. Revisión actual y puesta al día. *Cir. Esp.* **2005**, *77*, 6–17. [CrossRef]
4. Verwaal, V.J.; Bruin, S.; Boot, H.; van Slooten, G.; van Tinteren, H. 8-year follow-up of randomized trial: Cytoreduction and hyperthermic intraperitoneal chemotherapy versus systemic chemotherapy in patients with peritoneal carcinomatosis of colorectal cancer. *Ann. Surg. Oncol.* **2008**, *15*, 2426–2432. [CrossRef] [PubMed]
5. Elias, D.; Goere, D.; Dumont, F.; Honore, C.; Dartigues, P.; Stoclin, A.; Malka, D.; Boige, V.; Ducreux, M. Role of hyperthermic intraoperative peritoneal chemotherapy in the management of peritoneal metastases. *Eur. J. Cancer* **2014**, *50*, 332–340. [CrossRef]
6. Neuwirth, M.G.; Alexander, H.R.; Karakousis, G.C. Then and now: Cytoreductive surgery with hyperthermic intraperitoneal chemotherapy (HIPEC), a historical perspective. *J. Gastrointest. Oncol.* **2016**, *7*, 18. [CrossRef]
7. Sadeghi, B.; Arvieux, C.; Glehen, O.; Beaujard, A.C.; Rivoire, M.; Baulieux, J.; Fontaumard, E.; Brachet, A.; Caillot, J.L.; Faure, J.L.; et al. Peritoneal carcinomatosis from non-gynecologic malignancies: Results of the EVOCAPE 1 multicentric prospective study. *Cancer* **2000**, *88*, 358–363. [CrossRef]
8. Goere, D.; Passot, G.; Gelli, M.; Levine, E.A.; Bartlett, D.L.; Sugarbaker, P.H.; Glehen, O. Complete cytoreductive surgery plus HIPEC for peritoneal metastases from unusual cancer sites of origin: Results from a worldwide analysis issue of the Peritoneal Surface Oncology Group International (PSOGI). *Int. J. Hyperth.* **2017**, *33*, 520–527. [CrossRef]
9. Esquivel, J.; Sticca, R.; Sugarbaker, P.; Levine, E.; Yan, T.D.; Alexander, R.; Baratti, D.; Bartlett, D.; Barone, R.; Barrios, P.; et al. Cytoreductive surgery and hyperthermic intraperitoneal chemotherapy in the management of peritoneal surface malignancies of colonic origin: A consensus statement. Society of Surgical Oncology. *Ann. Surg. Oncol.* **2007**, *14*, 128–133. [CrossRef]
10. Glehen, O.; Kwiatkowski, F.; Sugarbaker, P.H.; Elias, D.; Levine, E.A.; De Simone, M.; Barone, R.; Yonemura, Y.; Cavaliere, F.; Quenet, F.; et al. Cytoreductive surgery combined with perioperative intraperitoneal chemotherapy for the management of peritoneal carcinomatosis from colorectal cancer: A multi-institutional study. *J. Clin. Oncol.* **2004**, *22*, 3284–3292. [CrossRef]
11. Elias, D.; Lefevre, J.H.; Chevalier, J.; Brouquet, A.; Marchal, F.; Classe, J.M.; Ferron, G.; Guilloit, J.M.; Meeus, P.; Goere, D.; et al. Complete cytoreductive surgery plus intraperitoneal chemohyperthermia with oxaliplatin for peritoneal carcinomatosis of colorectal origin. *J. Clin. Oncol.* **2009**, *27*, 681–685. [CrossRef] [PubMed]
12. Yang, X.J.; Huang, C.Q.; Suo, T.; Mei, L.J.; Yang, G.L.; Cheng, F.L.; Zhou, Y.F.; Xiong, B.; Yonemura, Y.; Li, Y. Cytoreductive surgery and hyperthermic intraperitoneal chemotherapy improves survival of patients with peritoneal carcinomatosis from gastric cancer: Final results of a phase III randomized clinical trial. *Ann. Surg. Oncol.* **2011**, *18*, 1575–1581. [CrossRef]
13. Yan, T.D.; Black, D.; Sugarbaker, P.H.; Zhu, J.; Yonemura, Y.; Petrou, G.; Morris, D.L. A systematic review and meta-analysis of the randomized controlled trials on adjuvant intraperitoneal chemotherapy for resectable gastric cancer. *Ann. Surg. Oncol.* **2007**, *14*, 2702–2713. [CrossRef] [PubMed]
14. Hotopp, T. HIPEC and CRS in peritoneal metastatic gastric cancer-who really benefits? *Surg. Oncol.* **2019**, *28*, 159–166. [CrossRef] [PubMed]
15. Manzanedo, I.; Pereira, F.; Rihuete-Caro, C.; Perez-Viejo, E.; Serrano, A.; Calvo, A.G.; Regueira, F.M.; Casado-Adam, A.; Cascales-Campos, P.A.; Arteaga, X.; et al. Cytoreductive Surgery and Hyperthermic Intraperitoneal Chemotherapy (HIPEC) for Gastric Cancer with Peritoneal Carcinomatosis: Multicenter Study of Spanish Group of Peritoneal Oncologic Surgery (GECOP). *Ann. Surg. Oncol.* **2019**, *26*, 2615–2621. [CrossRef]
16. Deraco, M.; Sinukumar, S.; Salcedo-Hernandez, R.A.; Rajendra, V.J.; Baratti, D.; Guaglio, M.; Nizri, E.; Kusamura, S. Clinico-pathological outcomes after total parietal peritonectomy, cytoreductive surgery and hyperthermic intraperitoneal chemotherapy in advanced serous papillary peritoneal carcinoma submitted to neoadjuvant systemic chemotherapy- largest single institute experience. *Eur. J. Surg. Oncol.* **2019**, *45*, 2103–2108. [CrossRef] [PubMed]
17. Sugarbaker, P.H. Peritonectomy procedures. *Ann. Surg.* **1995**, *221*, 29–42. [CrossRef]
18. Ozcelik, M.; Oyman, A.; Cil, I.; Duzgun, O.; Ozkan, O.F.; Ayhan, M. Cytoreductive Surgery versus Systemic Chemotherapy alone in Isolated Peritoneal Carcinomatosis of Colorectal Origin. *J. Coll. Physicians Surg. Pak.* **2021**, *31*, 1308–1313. [CrossRef]
19. Lei, Z.; Wang, Y.; Wang, J.; Wang, K.; Tian, J.; Zhao, Y.; Chen, L.; Wang, J.; Luo, J.; Jia, M.; et al. Evaluation of Cytoreductive Surgery With or Without Hyperthermic Intraperitoneal Chemotherapy for Stage III Epithelial Ovarian Cancer. *JAMA Netw. Open* **2020**, *3*, e2013940. [CrossRef]
20. Klaver, Y.L.; Hendriks, T.; Lomme, R.M.; Rutten, H.J.; Bleichrodt, R.P.; de Hingh, I.H. Intraoperative hyperthermic intraperitoneal chemotherapy after cytoreductive surgery for peritoneal carcinomatosis in an experimental model. *Br. J. Surg.* **2010**, *97*, 1874–1880. [CrossRef]

21. Bushati, M.; Rovers, K.P.; Sommariva, A.; Sugarbaker, P.H.; Morris, D.L.; Yonemura, Y.; Quadros, C.A.; Somashekhar, S.P.; Ceelen, W.; Dube, P.; et al. The current practice of cytoreductive surgery and HIPEC for colorectal peritoneal metastases: Results of a worldwide web-based survey of the Peritoneal Surface Oncology Group International (PSOGI). *Eur. J. Surg. Oncol.* **2018**, *44*, 1942–1948. [CrossRef]
22. Glehen, O.; Cotte, E.; Kusamura, S.; Deraco, M.; Baratti, D.; Passot, G.; Beaujard, A.C.; Noel, G.F. Hyperthermic intraperitoneal chemotherapy: Nomenclature and modalities of perfusion. *J. Surg. Oncol.* **2008**, *98*, 242–246. [CrossRef] [PubMed]
23. Sánchez-García, S.; Padilla-Valverde, D.; Villarejo-Campos, P.; Martín-Fernández, J.; García-Rojo, M.; Rodríguez-Martínez, M. Experimental development of an intra-abdominal chemohyperthermia model using a closed abdomen technique and a PRS-1.0 Combat CO2 recirculation system. *Surgery* **2014**, *155*, 719–725. [CrossRef] [PubMed]
24. Soriano, R.M.; Cascales-Campos, P.A.; Gil Martinez, J. *Cirugía de la Carcinomatosis Peritoneal*, 1st ed.; Cirujanos, A.E.D., Ed.; ARÁN EDICIONES SL: Madrid, Spain, 2018; Volume 6, p. 114.
25. Yonemura, Y.; Bandou, E.; Kawamura, T.; Endou, Y.; Sasaki, T. Quantitative prognostic indicators of peritoneal dissemination of gastric cancer. *Eur. J. Surg. Oncol.* **2006**, *32*, 602–606. [CrossRef] [PubMed]
26. Harmon, R.L.; Sugarbaker, P.H. Prognostic indicators in peritoneal carcinomatosis from gastrointestinal cancer. *Int. Semin. Surg. Oncol.* **2005**, *2*, 3. [CrossRef]
27. Glehen, O.; Gilly, F.N. Quantitative prognostic indicators of peritoneal surface malignancy: Carcinomatosis, sarcomatosis, and peritoneal mesothelioma. *Surg. Oncol. Clin. N. Am.* **2003**, *12*, 649–671. [CrossRef]
28. Younan, R.; Kusamura, S.; Baratti, D.; Cloutier, A.S.; Deraco, M. Morbidity, toxicity, and mortality classification systems in the local regional treatment of peritoneal surface malignancy. *J. Surg. Oncol.* **2008**, *98*, 253–257. [CrossRef]
29. Sugarbaker, P.H.; Alderman, R.; Edwards, G.; Marquardt, C.E.; Gushchin, V.; Esquivel, J.; Chang, D. Prospective morbidity and mortality assessment of cytoreductive surgery plus perioperative intraperitoneal chemotherapy to treat peritoneal dissemination of appendiceal mucinous malignancy. *Ann. Surg. Oncol.* **2006**, *13*, 635–644. [CrossRef]
30. Elias, D.; Gilly, F.; Boutitie, F.; Quenet, F.; Bereder, J.M.; Mansvelt, B.; Lorimier, G.; Dube, P.; Glehen, O. Peritoneal colorectal carcinomatosis treated with surgery and perioperative intraperitoneal chemotherapy: Retrospective analysis of 523 patients from a multicentric French study. *J. Clin. Oncol.* **2010**, *28*, 63–68. [CrossRef]
31. Glehen, O.; Osinsky, D.; Cotte, E.; Kwiatkowski, F.; Freyer, G.; Isaac, S.; Trillet-Lenoir, V.; Sayag-Beaujard, A.; François, Y.; Vignal, J. Intraperitoneal chemohyperthermia using a closed abdominal procedure and cytoreductive surgery for the treatment of peritoneal carcinomatosis: Morbidity and mortality analysis of 216 consecutive procedures. *Ann. Surg. Oncol.* **2003**, *10*, 863–869. [CrossRef]
32. Kusamura, S.; Younan, R.; Baratti, D.; Costanzo, P.; Favaro, M.; Gavazzi, C.; Deraco, M. Cytoreductive surgery followed by intraperitoneal hyperthermic perfusion: Analysis of morbidity and mortality in 209 peritoneal surface malignancies treated with closed abdomen technique. *Cancer* **2006**, *106*, 1144–1153. [CrossRef] [PubMed]
33. Levine, E.A.; Stewart, J.H.t.; Russell, G.B.; Geisinger, K.R.; Loggie, B.L.; Shen, P. Cytoreductive surgery and intraperitoneal hyperthermic chemotherapy for peritoneal surface malignancy: Experience with 501 procedures. *J. Am. Coll. Surg.* **2007**, *204*, 943–953; discussion 953–945. [CrossRef] [PubMed]
34. Sánchez-García, S.; Villarejo-Campos, P.; Padilla-Valverde, D.; Amo-Salas, M.; Martín-Fernández, J. Intraperitoneal chemotherapy hyperthermia (HIPEC) for peritoneal carcinomatosis of ovarian cancer origin by fluid and CO2 recirculation using the closed abdomen technique (PRS-1.0 Combat): A clinical pilot study. *Int. J. Hyperth.* **2016**, *32*, 488–495. [CrossRef]
35. Cianci, S.; Abatini, C.; Fagotti, A.; Chiofalo, B.; Tropea, A.; Biondi, A.; Scambia, G.; Pacelli, F. Hyperthermic intraperitoneal chemotherapy (HIPEC) for peritoneal malignancies using new hybrid CO_2 system: Preliminary experience in referral center. *Updat. Surg.* **2019**, *71*, 555–560. [CrossRef] [PubMed]
36. Mehta, A.; Hoven, J.V.D.; Rosing, H.; Hillebrand, M.; Nuijen, B.; Huitema, A.; Beijnen, J.; Verwaal, V. Stability of oxaliplatin in chloride-containing carrier solutions used in hyperthermic intraperitoneal chemotherapy. *Int. J. Pharm.* **2015**, *479*, 23–27. [CrossRef]
37. Pelz, J.O.; Stojadinovic, A.; Nissan, A.; Hohenberger, W.; Esquivel, J. Evaluation of a peritoneal surface disease severity score in patients with colon cancer with peritoneal carcinomatosis. *J. Surg. Oncol.* **2009**, *99*, 9–15. [CrossRef] [PubMed]
38. Glehen, O.; Gilly, F.N.; Arvieux, C.; Cotte, E.; Boutitie, F.; Mansvelt, B.; Bereder, J.M.; Lorimier, G.; Quenet, F.; Elias, D.; et al. Peritoneal carcinomatosis from gastric cancer: A multi-institutional study of 159 patients treated by cytoreductive surgery combined with perioperative intraperitoneal chemotherapy. *Ann. Surg. Oncol.* **2010**, *17*, 2370–2377. [CrossRef] [PubMed]
39. Yan, T.D.; Black, D.; Savady, R.; Sugarbaker, P.H. Systematic review on the efficacy of cytoreductive surgery combined with perioperative intraperitoneal chemotherapy for peritoneal carcinomatosis from colorectal carcinoma. *J. Clin. Oncol.* **2006**, *24*, 4011–4019. [CrossRef] [PubMed]
40. Quenet, F.; Elias, D.; Roca, L.; Goere, D.; Ghouti, L.; Pocard, M.; Facy, O.; Arvieux, C.; Lorimier, G.; Pezet, D. A UNICANCER phase III trial of hyperthermic intra-peritoneal chemotherapy (HIPEC) for colorectal peritoneal carcinomatosis (PC): PRODIGE 7. *J. Clin. Oncol.* **2018**, *36*, 3503. [CrossRef]
41. Beaujard, A.C.; Glehen, O.; Caillot, J.L.; Francois, Y.; Bienvenu, J.; Panteix, G.; Garbit, F.; Grandclement, E.; Vignal, J.; Gilly, F.N. Intraperitoneal chemohyperthermia with mitomycin C for digestive tract cancer patients with peritoneal carcinomatosis. *Cancer* **2000**, *88*, 2512–2519. [CrossRef]

42. Quénet, F. Colorectal peritoneal carcinomatosis: What is the future of HIPEC? *Eur. J. Surg. Oncol.* **2018**, *44*, 1847–1848. [CrossRef] [PubMed]
43. Klaver, C.E.; Groenen, H.; Morton, D.G.; Laurberg, S.; Bemelman, W.A.; Tanis, P.J. The research committee of the European Society of Coloproctology Recommendations and consensus on the treatment of peritoneal metastases of colorectal origin: A systematic review of national and international guidelines. *Color. Dis.* **2017**, *19*, 224–236. [CrossRef] [PubMed]
44. Aoyagi, T.; Terracina, K.P.; Raza, A.; Takabe, K. Current treatment options for colon cancer peritoneal carcinomatosis. *World J. Gastroenterol.* **2014**, *20*, 12493–12500. [CrossRef]
45. Sanchez-Garcia, S.; Padilla-Valverde, D.; Villarejo-Campos, P.; Garcia-Santos, E.P.; Martin-Fernandez, J. Hyperthermic chemotherapy intra-abdominal laparoscopic approach: Development of a laparoscopic model using CO2 recirculation system and clinical translation in peritoneal carcinomatosis. *Int. J. Hyperth.* **2017**, *33*, 684–689. [CrossRef] [PubMed]
46. Van der Speeten, K.; Stuart, O.A.; Sugarbaker, P.H. Pharmacokinetics and pharmacodynamics of perioperative cancer chemotherapy in peritoneal surface malignancy. *Cancer J.* **2009**, *15*, 216–224. [CrossRef] [PubMed]
47. Sugarbaker, P. Laboratory and clinical basis for hyperthermia as a component of intracavitary chemotherapy. *Int. J. Hyperth.* **2007**, *23*, 431–442. [CrossRef]
48. Armour, E.P.; McEachern, D.; Wang, Z.; Corry, P.M.; Martinez, A. Sensitivity of human cells to mild hyperthermia. *Cancer Res.* **1993**, *53*, 2740–2744. [PubMed]
49. Issels, R.D. Hyperthermia adds to chemotherapy. *Eur. J. Cancer* **2008**, *44*, 2546–2554. [CrossRef]
50. Pelz, J.O.; Vetterlein, M.; Grimmig, T.; Kerscher, A.G.; Moll, E.; Lazariotou, M.; Matthes, N.; Faber, M.; Germer, C.T.; Waaga-Gasser, A.M.; et al. Hyperthermic intraperitoneal chemotherapy in patients with peritoneal carcinomatosis: Role of heat shock proteins and dissecting effects of hyperthermia. *Ann. Surg. Oncol.* **2013**, *20*, 1105–1113. [CrossRef] [PubMed]
51. Kusamura, S.; Dominique, E.; Baratti, D.; Younan, R.; Deraco, M. Drugs, carrier solutions and temperature in hyperthermic intraperitoneal chemotherapy. *J. Surg. Oncol.* **2008**, *98*, 247–252. [CrossRef] [PubMed]
52. Yonemura, Y.; de Aretxabala, X.; Fujimura, T.; Fushida, S.; Katayama, K.; Bandou, E.; Sugiyama, K.; Kawamura, T.; Kinoshita, K.; Endou, Y.; et al. Intraoperative chemohyperthermic peritoneal perfusion as an adjuvant to gastric cancer: Final results of a randomized controlled study. *Hepatogastroenterology* **2001**, *48*, 1776–1782. [PubMed]
53. Esquis, P.; Consolo, D.; Magnin, G.; Pointaire, P.; Moretto, P.; Ynsa, M.D.; Beltramo, J.L.; Drogoul, C.; Simonet, M.; Benoit, L.; et al. High intra-abdominal pressure enhances the penetration and antitumor effect of intraperitoneal cisplatin on experimental peritoneal carcinomatosis. *Ann. Surg.* **2006**, *244*, 106–112. [CrossRef] [PubMed]
54. Elias, D.; Benizri, E.; Di Pietrantonio, D.; Menegon, P.; Malka, D.; Raynard, B. Comparison of two kinds of intraperitoneal chemotherapy following complete cytoreductive surgery of colorectal peritoneal carcinomatosis. *Ann. Surg. Oncol.* **2007**, *14*, 509–514. [CrossRef] [PubMed]

Journal of
Clinical Medicine

MDPI

Review

Development of the Peritoneal Metastasis: A Review of Back-Grounds, Mechanisms, Treatments and Prospects

Kaijie Ren [1,†], Xin Xie [2,†], Tianhao Min [1], Tuanhe Sun [1], Haonan Wang [1], Yong Zhang [1], Chengxue Dang [1,*] and Hao Zhang [1,*]

[1] Department of Surgical Oncology, The First Affiliated Hospital of Xi'an Jiaotong University, Xi'an 710061, China

[2] Department of Nuclear Medicine, The First Affiliated Hospital of Xi'an Jiaotong University, Xi'an 710061, China

* Correspondence: dangchengxue@mail.xjtu.edu.cn (C.D.); hao.zhang@mail.xjtu.edu.cn (H.Z.); Tel.: +86-13319202569 (C.D.); +86-13571946099 (H.Z.)

† These authors contribute equally to this study.

Abstract: Peritoneal metastasis is a malignant disease which originated from several gastrointestinal and gynecological carcinomas and has been leading to a suffering condition in patients for decades. Currently, as people have gradually become more aware of the severity of peritoneal carcinomatosis, new molecular mechanisms for targeting and new treatments have been proposed. However, due to the uncertainty of influencing factors involved and a lack of a standardized procedure for this treatment, as well as a need for more clinical data for specific evaluation, more research is needed, both for preventing and treating. We aim to summarize backgrounds, mechanisms and treatments in this area and conclude limitations or new aspects for treatments.

Keywords: peritoneal carcinomatosis; molecular mechanisms; treatment

1. Introduction

Peritoneal metastasis refers to the development and spread of several gastrointestinal and gynecological carcinomas in the peritoneal cavity; related carcinomas include colorectal carcinoma, gastric carcinoma, ovarian carcinoma, etc. [1]. There are other primary peritoneal tumors, which mostly originated from mesothelium, such as serous carcinoma, malignant mesothelioma and pseudomyxoma peritonei. Nearly all types are similar in presentation, diagnosis, evaluation and treatment [2,3].

The occurrence of peritoneal metastasis has been indicated to significantly decrease overall survival in patients with gastrointestinal cancer. Due to the lack of effective systemic chemotherapy, peritoneal metastasis is mostly considered a terminal condition. A study from France collected data from 1976 to 2012 for 9148 patients with colorectal adenocarcinoma and indicated that the proportions of patients who underwent curative resection for synchronous and metachronous peritoneal carcinomatosis were 11% and 9%, respectively, and these patients had 3-year overall survival rates of 8% and 5% [4]. Additionally, patients with peritoneal metastasis are more likely to relapse than those with single tumors, regardless of what methods were used during treatment [5]; however, active treatment still prolongs overall survival [6].

In the last century, peritoneal metastasis was treated as a terminal and uncurable condition, but treatment advances, especially cytoreductive surgery (CRS) and hyperthermic intraperitoneal chemotherapy (HIPEC), have improved the life quality of patients; thus, the outcomes of peritoneal carcinomatosis have been changed [7]. Currently, several new methods, such as pressurized intraperitoneal aerosol chemotherapy, new delivery systems targeting local regions and molecular targeted drugs, have been proposed. A few phase II and phase III studies have investigated the effects of multimodal approaches and are still ongoing. The aim of this review was to acknowledge widely accepted concepts of peritoneal carcinomatosis, summarize the physiology and pathophysiology of this disease and assess new treatments for peritoneal carcinomatosis to have a better understanding of this condition.

2. Physiology and Function of the Peritoneum

The peritoneum, as a serous membrane, consists of a monolayer of mesothelial cells connected to a basement membrane on a layer of connective tissue. The submesothelial layer consists of the extracellular matrix, which is composed of multiple types of collagens, glycoproteins, glycosaminoglycans and proteoglycans. Mesothelial cells are present in a single layer and generally show a flattened, stretched, squamous or cuboidal appearance. Different types of mesothelial cells are present at different positions and show various functions. Mesothelial cells with cuboidal shapes are found mostly at the visceral peritoneum; compared to cells with other shapes, these cells contain rougher endoplasmic reticulum and Golgi apparatus organelles, microtubules, intracellular vesicles and microfilaments, indicating their good biosynthetic capacity and active transmembrane transport. Vascular structures and lymphatic systems are present in the subserous space [8].

The peritoneum allows the exchange of molecules and the production and transportation of peritoneal fluid, which provides a suitable environment for intra-abdominal organs. Recently, other functions of the peritoneum have been found, including glycosaminoglycan and surfactant secretion, inflammation inhibition, leucocyte migration, antigen presentation and tissue repair. Functional peritoneal cells are vital in maintaining peritoneum homeostasis. Its role in tumor dissemination has also been studied due to the secretion of growth factors and the presence of specific structures, such as milky spots [9].

Milky spots, which are submesothelial lymphoid structures, are found in the peritoneum, especially in the omentum. Milky spots consist of aggregates of mesenchymal cells surrounding capillary convolutions, mostly macrophages, lymphocytes, type 2 innate lymphoid cells (ILC2s) and $CXCL13^+/FDCM1^+$ stromal cells [10]. In recent studies, milky spots were found to be linked to tumor metastasis, indicating that more attention should be given to peritoneal carcinomatosis.

3. Peritoneal Metastasis

Peritoneal metastasis occurs via multiple ways. Usually, gastrointestinal (bowel wall penetration in cases of colorectal cancer) and gynecological carcinomas could directly implant cancer cells into the peritoneum, or via lymphatic ways, either due to a full-thickness invasion of the bowel wall of a primary tumor or blood and lymphatic vessels damage during a procedure. Other types of cancer, such as lung cancer, could occur through blood flow [1,11,12].

There are widely accepted steps in peritoneal metastasis. First, single cancer cells or clumps detach from the primary tumor and spread into the peritoneal cavity. Second, these cancer cells become susceptible to regular peritoneal transport along predictable routes. Third, these cells attach to and invade the distant peritoneum. Fourth, the cells invade the subperitoneal space. The underlying connective tissue provides the necessary scaffold for tumor proliferation. The final step involves angiogenesis, which sustains tumor proliferation and enables further growth [11] (Figure 1).

Single cancer cells or clumps detach from the primary tumor, spread into the peritoneal cavity and attach to the distant peritoneum; then, cancer cells invade the underlying connective tissue in different ways.

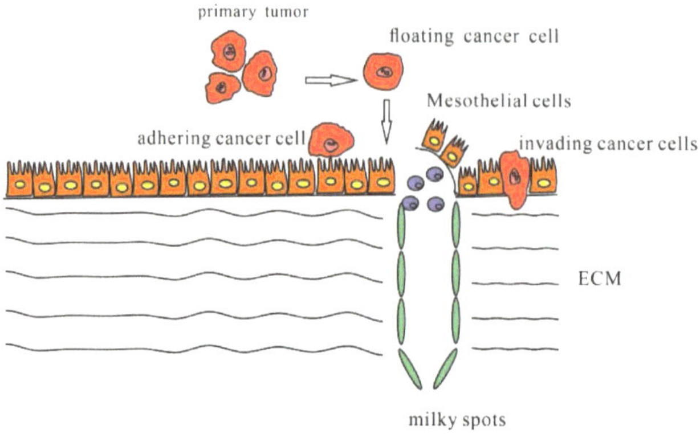

Figure 1. Steps of occurring peritoneal metastasis.

The detachment of tumor cells from the primary tumor could be spontaneous or secondary due to internal and external factors (mostly due to improper iatrogenic operation) [13]. Usually, high interstitial fluid pressure leads tumor cells to detach spontaneously due to rapid cell proliferation, high tumor blood vascular permeability, lack of functional lymphatic circulation, interstitial fibrosis and contraction of the interstitial matrix mediated by stromal fibroblasts [14]. However, it is interesting that performing laparoscopy did not seem to increase the risks occurring with peritoneal metastasis, leaving choices which are better for the outcomes of patients [15].

Once tumor cells detach from the primary tumor, they are mostly transplanted into four regions: the Pouch of Douglas at the rectosigmoid level, the right lower quadrant at the lower end of the small bowel mesentery, the left lower quadrant along the superior border of the sigmoid mesocolon and colon and the right paracolic gutter lateral to the cecum and ascending colon. The interaction of gravity, diaphragmatic excursion, mesenteric reflections and peritoneal recesses leads to flowing toward the pelvis and from the pelvis, along the right paracolic gutter, toward the subdiaphragmatic space [11].

It is worth noting that once tumor cells detach from the primary location, they must survive before they successfully metastases. Once cancer cells are in the peritoneal cavity, a change of the environment stimulated tumor cells, which favored their survival. Anoikis resistance is the most related phenotype that cancer cells develop which grants their ability to survive in the peritoneal cavity. There are ways tumor cells escape death and develop anoikis resistance, including modifying surface molecules, regulation of activating pathways and other mechanisms. For example, several transcription factors and genes are activated in gastric cancer cells; nuclear MTH9-VTNNB1, TCF7L2-PLAUR and NOX4-EGFR/ROS could promote anoikis resistance [16–18]. Another mechanism is that the activation of Integrins have been found to be participating in metastasis in ovarian cancer; integrin $\alpha 5\beta 3$ sustained cell survival and resisted anoikis by activating transcription of Bcl-2 [19]. The integrins also protected gastric cancer cells from anoikis as well [20]. Furthermore, upregulating KRAS and MEK-ERK in ovarian cancer cells could stabilize spheroid formation; in this form, it has advantages in promoting survival and metastasis than single cells, and tumor-associated macrophages also involved in spheroid formation, by promoting binding of cancer cells and activating EGFR signaling pathways [21,22]. In all, cancer cells must achieve certain molecular changes so that they can survive once they detach from the primary tumor, which explains why a high expression of some molecules, for example, CXCR4 in gastric cancer, have a higher rate of peritoneal metastasis occurring [23].

Peritoneal cells are essential in occurring metastasis by interacting with cancer cells in multiple ways: direct physical contact, soluble cytokines in microenvironment regulation by paracrine activities or reaction with a matrix, such as ECM components. There are mainly several mechanisms in peritoneal metastasis. Several types of cancer cells could induce apoptosis of peritoneal mesothelial cells, causing a breach onto the peritoneum, which will be mentioned below. Usually, an inflammatory environment would cause peritoneal cells to produce cytokines and adhesion molecules, resulting in peritoneal metastasis. TGF-beta secreted by gastric cancer cells was studied to induce changes of mesothelial cell morphology, leading to peritoneal fibrosis, or changing into fibroblast phenotype, ending in peritoneal metastasis [24–26].

Senescent peritoneal mesothelial cells are found to promote peritoneal metastasis. SASP, senescence-associated secretory phenotype, refers to several highly secreted cytokines (e.g., IL-1, IL-6, IL-13, IL-15), chemokines (e.g., CXCL1, CXCL8, CXCL12, ENA-78), growth factors (e.g., EGF, FGF, HGF, TGF-β, VEGF, angiogenin, epiregulin), extracellular matrix (ECM) proteins and remodeling enzymes (e.g., MMP-1, -3, -10), soluble receptors and ligands (e.g., ICAM-1, EGF-R, Fas) and other elements that promote cancer proliferation and metastases [27].

Malignant ascites is a lipid-rich microenvironment, mostly from differentiated preadipocytes stimulated by cancer cells. These cells mature and release free fatty acids, therefore enhancing cancer cell proliferation and EMT. Cancer cells in ascites also tend to produce more enzymes from fatty acid metabolism, with enhanced fatty acid oxidation, promoting peritoneal metastasis [28,29].

Adhesion and invasion into the peritoneum involve multiple molecular mechanisms facilitating cancer cell metastasis (Figure 2). These cells could directly adhere to the peritoneum and invade the submesothelial tissue, or cells could travel through milky spots. Although the immune function of milky spots is important for the defense against microorganisms, they are involved in a pathway for peritoneal carcinomatosis [30]. Milky spots usually provide a microenvironment suitable for cancer cells to implant and grow. Several studies have investigated how gastric cancer cells are implanted and transferred through milky spots: they provide a hypoxic microenvironment for gastric cancer cells to implant and grow, and HIF-1α in the microenvironment plays a significant role during progression. Hypoxia could also induce the EMT of gastric cancer cells [31]. Macrophages in milky spots produce MDC/CCL22 and its receptor CCR4, which are highly expressed in the omentum and the diaphragm underlining, contributing to gastric cancer cell survival and growth [32].

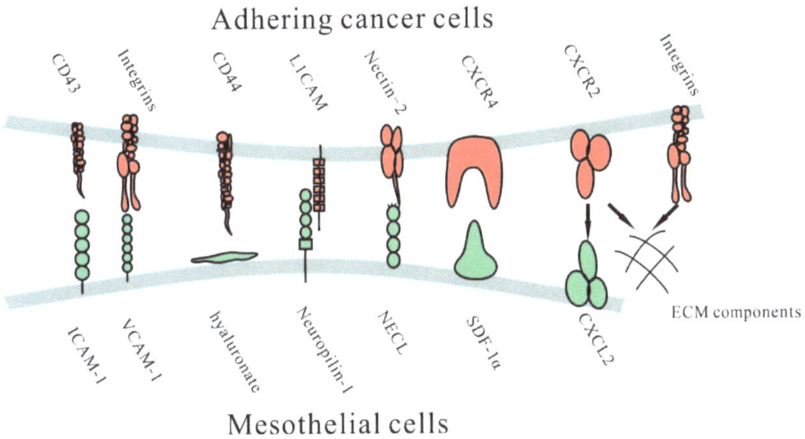

Figure 2. Molecular mechanisms of adhesive interactions mediating peritoneal carcinomatosis. ICAM-1 = intercellular adhesion molecule-1. VCAM-1= vascular cell adhesion molecule-1. L1CAM = L1 cell adhesion molecule. NECL = Nectin-like (NECL) family. CD44 = hyalonurate receptor. SDF-1α = stromal cell-derived factor 1α. CXCR4 = CXC receptor 4. CXCR2 = CXC receptor 2. CXCL12 = CXC ligand 12.

3.1. Adhesion to the Peritoneum

Once tumor cells detach from the primary tumor, they float in the peritoneal fluid and travel until they contact the peritoneum. Adhesion of free cancer cells to the peritoneal surface relies on several adhesion molecular mechanisms, such as several integrins, proteoglycans and the immunoglobulin superfamily.

3.1.1. Immunoglobulin Superfamily

The immunoglobulin superfamily is a group of cell adhesion molecules, including ICAM-1, VCAM-1 and L1CAM. Intercellular adhesion molecule-1 (ICAM-1) is a surface molecule expressed by mesothelial cells, cancer cells and endothelial cells [33]. It was found that it could enhance tumor cell adhesion mediated by IL-6 or TNF-α [33]. However, Hiroaki et al. indicated that ICAM-1 could reduce lymph node metastasis, which left the specific effect of ICAM-1 in peritoneal metastasis unknown [34].

Vascular cell adhesion molecule-1 (VCAM-1) is a known, highly expressed membrane protein on mesothelial cells and has been found to play a role in adhesion to the peritoneum in ovarian cancer [35]. A current study found that VCAM-1 was related to clinicopathological factors in colorectal cancer, such as lymph node metastasis and clinical stage [36], suggesting that it might play a role in multiple types of cancer.

L1 cell adhesion molecule (L1CAM), an important molecule and marker found in ovarian cancer for poor prognosis, has been found to be related to adhesion and invasion, and an antibody against L1CAM could significantly suppress this progression [37]. It is also involved in the metastatic process in gastric cancer, predicting metastasis-related clinicopathological features and unfavorable outcomes, and could be a feasible predictor of oncological outcome [38].

Studies have found that nectin-2, an adhesion molecule participating in cell proliferation, differentiation and migration of epithelial, endothelial, immune and nervous cells, is associated with tumor growth, adhesion and angiogenesis in ovarian cancer [39]. It was found to be significantly upregulated in patients who had lymph node metastasis or residual tumors >1 cm after surgery, as well as in samples of tumor tissues and lesions on the peritoneum, which suggest its role in metastasis of ovarian cancer [40].

3.1.2. Proteoglycans

CD44, a cell-surface proteoglycan, participates in behaviors such as cell interaction, adhesion and migration. It is overexpressed in gastrointestinal and gynecological cancers [41]. Specifically, several studies found that CD44 partly mediates adhesion, such as that exhibited by cancer cells attaching to peritoneal mesothelial cells [42]. CD44-mediated adhesion could also partly explain metastasis in the inflammatory microenvironment after surgery, in which several cytokines, such as TGF-β1, IL-1b and TNF-α, are generated, resulting in upregulated CD44 expression [43].

3.1.3. Integrins

Integrins are a superfamily of cell adhesion receptors consisting of 24 members, each of which is composed of α and β subunits, and recently, integrins participating in cancer metastasis have been investigated [44]. Studies have found that integrin $\alpha 2\beta 1$ participates in the peritoneal metastasis. Furthermore, it is a potential target for the treatment of peritoneal metastasis [45]. Integrin $\alpha 3\beta 1$ was also found to be involved in the adherence of gastric cancer cells to the peritoneum [46]. Integrin $\alpha 4\beta 1$ partly mediated peritoneal metastasis of ovarian cancer; furthermore, antibodies against it could increase ovarian cancer response to carboplatin, while treating with antibodies alone showed no response [47]. This phenomenon shows potential in clinical use.

Due to the hypoxic microenvironment, SIRT1 is degraded via the autophagic lysosomal pathway, causing increased acetylation of HIF-1α and secretion of VEGFA. Under these conditions, VEGFA derived from peritoneal mesothelial cells acts on VEGFR1 in gastric cancer cells, increasing integrin α5 and fibronectin expression, causing further adhesion to the peritoneum [48].

3.1.4. CXC Subfamily

SDF-1α is a chemokine of the CXC subfamily on mesothelial cells. Its upregulation was indicated to possibly be due to bioactive cytokines secreted from tumor cells and was found to be associated with enhanced intraperitoneal dissemination of epithelial ovarian carcinoma cells. Another possible mechanism is that CXCR2 secreted by CT-26 colon cancer cells could induce cell proliferation and migration by combining with CXCL2 on ECM components, blocking this process inhibited cell proliferation and migration [49].

3.1.5. Other Molecules

Wnt5a is a noncanonical Wnt ligand that is highly expressed in ascites in female patients with ovarian cancer and promotes ovarian tumor cell adhesion, migration and invasion. The downstream effector is the Src family kinase Fgr, which is a potential target for the treatment of ovarian cancer [50]. Other molecules are being investigated for possible treatment.

Currently, there are various molecules in research connecting adhesion to peritoneum, and several of them showed the possibilities of predicting outcomes or providing treatment opinions. Whether those mechanisms could be used in vivo, and their effect, is still in need of investigation.

3.2. *Invasion into the Peritoneum*

After adhesion, tumor cells need to invade the submesothelial tissue to achieve colonization; this process could be adhering to the ECM through the gap between mesothelial cells or directly induce mesothelial cell apoptosis. Carbon dioxide pneumoperitoneum temporarily enlarges intercellular clefts and exposes the ECM, allowing tumor cells to access the ECM more easily by using RGD peptides or pseudo-RGD peptides [51]. Tumor cells could also directly influence the function of mesothelial cells. Heath et al. found that SW480 colorectal cancer cells could induce FAS-dependent apoptosis of cultured human mesothelial cells and that tumor–mesothelial adhesion was essential for inducing apoptosis. This study suggested that this phenomenon plays a role in peritoneal carcinomatosis [52].

Several studies have shown that matrix metalloproteinases (MMPs) contribute to the invasion of the submesothelial tissue by causing degradation of the ECM and contraction of mesothelial cells. MMPs are a family of zinc-dependent endopeptidases that are involved in the degradation of various proteins in the extracellular matrix (ECM). Their functions in cancer invasion and metastasis have been found gradually. MMP-7 is likely to be associated with adhesion, as the downregulation of MMP-7 could suppress invasion without influencing proliferation; it also takes part in serosal involvement, lymph node metastasis, poor differentiation of cancer and peritoneal dissemination, indicating its role in peritoneal adhesion [53]. Another matrix metalloproteinase is MMP-9. In vitro studies have shown that peritoneal mesothelial cells can also secrete MMP-9 under TNF-α stimulation in gastric cancer cells, which enhances cancer cell invasion [54]. MMP2/9 were found strongly upregulated in colon tumor tissues, and inhibition of them could reduce colonization [55].

4. Diagnosis and Evaluation of Peritoneal Metastasis

The diagnosis of peritoneal carcinomatosis relies on imaging, biopsy and laparoscopy. CT and PET/CT are the most used methods for the detection of peritoneal metastasis; an enhanced CT scan could provide valuable information for metastasis detection [56], especially for pseudomyxoma peritonei [57]. PET/CT with radioisotopes is more sensitive for diagnosis than CT, according to Koh et al. [58]; however, other research found CT to be more sensitive than PET/CT for diagnosis [59]. PET is traditionally more sensitive to tumors with hypermetabolic uptake, but not minor nodules [58,60]. Diffusion-weighted (DW) MRI was another method and seemed to be the same as CT in sensitivity or PET/CT in diagnosis [61,62]. In addition, PET/CT appeared favorable in sensitivity as well, but showed weak ability in excluding diagnosis of peritoneal metastasis [63,64]. Imaging methods can assist in assessing peritoneal metastasis, thus evaluating if cytoreduction is possible. Compared with imaging, the most precise method of diagnosis is peritoneal visualization and biopsy, for example, exploratory laparotomy, but this approach is invasive [65]. It is worth noting that, recently, a fluorescent probe called gGlu-HMRG had been used to detect tiny tumors on the peritoneal wall, showing potential in both diagnosis and assistance for fluorescence-guided surgery for peritoneal carcinomatosis [66]. Currently, despite the limitations of CT, it is a still powerful and cost-effective tool for general metastasis detection, making it the first choice for detection and diagnosis; PET/CT and MRI could be used in an alternative way and in specific situations.

A way of evaluating peritoneal metastasis is using the peritoneal cancer index (PCI). PCI includes the surgical peritoneal cancer index (sPCI) and pathologic peritoneal index (pPCI), the former of which requires evaluating peritoneal metastasis during surgery. Surgeons record the number and size of lesions in each of the 13 peritoneal regions and add them to obtain the sPCI. The pPCI is scored through the pathologic evaluation of specimens. sPCI and pPCI do not always seem consistent, for the former is mostly subjective, though sPCI could provide valuable information for the evaluation of patients [67]. Though pPCI is more objective, specimens would shrink during the process, causing misjudgment of tumor size. Furthermore, there were no standard procedures for the evaluation of specimens from CRS, thus, further research needs to be conducted [68]. CT-PCI used a CT scan for the evaluation of the disease burden and prognosis, helping for these aspects, regardless of its accuracy [60,69].

It is also interesting to evaluate whether there were differences between primary tumors and metastasis tumors in molecular and gene expression to further understand the mechanisms of metastasis and to provide targeted treatment. Several studies found high consistency in colorectal cancer in both dMMR, MSI status and biomarkers [70,71]; however, there were other studies that found different expression in colorectal cancer between primary tumor and metastases, a significant enrichment for CMS4 in peritoneal metastasis, providing a possible treatment combined with CRS-HIPEC to reduce metastasis tumors [72]. Furthermore, different expressions or mutations were detected in gastric cancer based on a multi-omic profiling, suggesting a molecular-targeting therapy separate from therapy on primary tumors.

The differences of biomarkers between colorectal cancer and its metastases have been compared [73,74], including KRAS/BRAF mutation and MSI status, indicating the importance of testing mutations in peritoneal metastasis and treating methods. However, there is still in lack of research and data in the area, which suggests a further evaluation of personalized treatment.

5. Treatment to Peritoneal Metastasis

Peritoneal metastasis was traditionally considered a terminal condition and thus lacked effective treatment. However, several methods and ideas have been proposed and used in the clinic with exciting progress (Figure 3).

In surgery for primary tumors, traditional ways to reduce the incidence of peritoneal metastasis are to follow a no-touch isolation technique (NTIT)—complete removal of adjacent invaded structures and surgical margins deep in the healthy tissue—and other standard surgery procedures, which reduce the feasibility of surgery-induced local metastasis and blood metastasis [75]. However, recent clinical trials questioned the superiority of the NTIT [76], indicating that further treatments are needed.

Intraperitoneal chemotherapy has been widely applied, compared to systemic chemotherapy for peritoneal carcinomatosis, because not all reagents of systemically applied chemotherapy could be fully delivered to the peritoneum, possibly due to the peritoneum-plasma barrier. This barrier leads to peritoneal clearance being much slower than systemic clearance; thus, a high intraperitoneal chemotherapy dose would result in moderate systemic drug exposure [77].

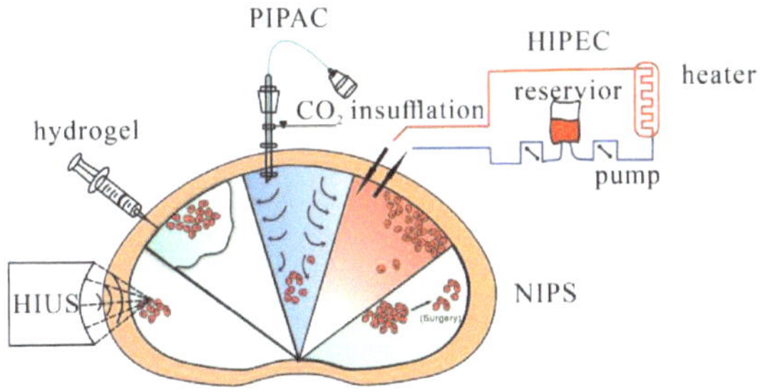

Figure 3. Treatments being applied to peritoneal metastasis. HIPEC = hyperthermic intraperitoneal chemotherapy. PIPAC = pressurized intraperitoneal aerosol chemotherapy. HIUS = high-intensity ultrasound. NIPS = neoadjuvant intraperitoneal and systemic chemotherapy. Hydrogel = using hydrogel as a delivery system for local regions.

HIPEC, known as hyperthermic intraperitoneal chemotherapy, uses specific chemical reagents and a high temperature to kill tumor cells. It has mainly been evaluated in peritoneal carcinomatosis in colorectal, mucinous appendicular adenocarcinoma and ovarian cancer [78–83]. The main advantage of HIPEC is the maintenance of a high regional reagent concentration, and blood drainage of the peritoneal surface occurs via the portal vein to the liver. Increasing the concentration in the liver would suppress liver metastasis as well. Another advantage is that 41–43 °C hyperthermia could directly kill tumor cells by inhibiting RNA synthesis and mitotic arrest and increasing the number of lysosomes and the activity of lysosomal enzymes. Heat also increases the cytotoxicity of certain chemotherapeutic drugs and enhances tissue penetration [84]. HIPEC is usually administered in the operating room immediately after CRS, due to limited drug penetration in tumor tissues, and is mainly used to kill microscopic residual disease after CRS.

However, due to the direct administration of drugs into the peritoneum, choices of these drugs must meet certain criteria. Typically, these reagents should be effective against malignant cells and low local toxicity after administration. Additionally, these reagents should be cycle-nonspecific and induce heat-synergized effects [84]. Specific reagent effects, toxicity to malignant cells and penetration into tumor tissues during systemic chemotherapy should be considered to determine which method is more effective. Reagents that require transformation into an active form in the liver should be excluded. In addition, the most important feature is that reagents should be slowly absorbed from the peritoneal cavity and rapidly cleared via hepatic and/or renal mechanisms so that a high concentration of drug can be maintained with low systemic toxicity [85].

Several studies have compared factors influencing the outcomes of CRS-HIPEC (Table 1). Though most studies used different strategies, the results suggested that a patient's survival was prolonged after a complete procedure. Factors involved in HIPEC include choices of drugs, applied dose, duration, carrier solution, perfusate volume, perfusate concentration and use of an open vs. closed technique [85]. Interestingly, repeated CRS-HIPECs seemed to be beneficial for patients occurring metastasis limited to peritoneum, suggesting that it might be suitable for specific patients to prolong survival [86]. However, HIPEC had risks of causing changes to genetic patterns between tumors and normal tissues and an upregulation of heat shock-related genes, to be specific, which would be an adverse effect, and an idea of combining other treatments [87].

Table 1. Different studies of HIPEC in different diseases.

Ref.	Disease	Type	Group	Survival	Death and Complication	Recurrence
Glehen [78]	colorectal cancer	retrospective multicenter study	506	overall median survival: 19.2 months complete CRS vs. not complete CRS: 32.4 months vs. 8.4 months ($p < 0.001$)	complication rate: 22.9% death rate: 4%	371 recurrence (73.3% with 158 (41.9%) peritoneal recurrence
Glehen [79]	colorectal cancer	retrospective study	53	median overall survival: 12.8 months CCR-0 vs. CCR-1 vs. CCR-2: 32.9 vs. 12.5 vs. 8.1 ($p < 0.001$)	complication rate: 23% death rate: 4%	–
Kecmanovic [80]	colorectal cancer	retrospective study	18	median overall survival: 15 months	complication: 8	3 live with cancer progress, 3 died of it
Rosa [81]	colorectal cancer	retrospective study	67	median overall survival: 41 months 3-year overall survival: 43%	complication rate: 35.8%	–
François Quénet [82]	colorectal cancer	PRODIGE 7 a multicenter, randomized, open-label, phase 3 trial	133 (CRS plus HIPEC) vs. 132(CRS)	median overall survival: 41.7 months (CRS plus HIPEC) vs. 41.2 months (CRS)		–
Driel [83]	ovarian cancer	a multicenter, open-label, phase 3 trial	123 (Surgery) vs. 122 (Surgery plus HIPEC)	median overall survival: 33.9 months (Surgery) vs. 45.7 months. (Surgery plus HIPEC) 3-year overall: 48% (Surgery) vs. 62% (Surgery plus HIPEC)	Complication: 122 (Surgery) vs. 118 (Surgery plus HIPEC) death: 62% (Surgery) vs. 50% (Surgery plus HIPEC)	recurrence or death: 89% (Surgery) vs. 81% (Surgery plus HIPEC)

CRS: cytoreductive surgery; CCR-0: complete resection; CCR-1: diameter of residual nodules 5 mm or less; CCR-2: diameter of residual nodules more than 5 mm; HIPEC: hyperthermic intraperitoneal chemotherapy.

Overall, most studies recommended that CRS-HIPEC could improve outcomes, with the restriction that low disease extent (limited peritoneal metastasis) and complete CRS indicated better outcomes, indicating its limitation in clinical use [88]. However, there is still a lack of researchers comparing different strategies and different factors of HIPEC, leading to uncertainty for specific treatment efficiency. Therefore, further research and new methods should be proposed and the advantages of different strategies for a limited number of procedures for different stages of peritoneal carcinomatosis, due to disadvantages, complications and limitations for CRS-HIPEC, should be compared, and personalized treatments should be provided in the future.

A new method called pressurized intraperitoneal aerosol chemotherapy (PIPAC) has been studied and brought to clinical use. Compared with systemic chemotherapy and chemical solutions administered to the peritoneal cavity, PIPAC could optimize the uniformity of chemical concentrations in the peritoneal cavity, enhance drug penetration by increasing intraperitoneal hydrostatic pressure against interstitial fluid pressure, limit blood outflow and adjust the environment of the peritoneal cavity, such as temperature and pH, to achieve better tissue targeting [89]. A cohort study investigated PIPAC combined with systemic chemotherapy to treat diffuse malignant peritoneal mesothelioma (DMPM). In this study, 26 patients with unresectable disease were treated with PIPAC, and 20 of them had not previously received CRS. An improvement of symptoms was reported for 32% of the patients, and control of ascites was reported in 46%. Fourteen of fifteen patients were treated with CRS plus HIPEC and achieved complete resection. The median overall survival period was 12 months, and the median progression-free survival (PFS) was significantly better among the patients who underwent resection than among those who did not (33.5 vs. 7.4 months, $p < 0.001$). This study demonstrated that for patients with unresectable DMPM, PIPAC could be used as neoadjuvant chemotherapy and increase the possibility for further CRS [90]. Alyami et al. found that unresectable peritoneal metastasis treated with repeated PIPAC could allow secondary treatment: CRS- HIPEC [91]. There are multiple studies which have evaluated the safety and feasibility of PIPAC combined with chemical drugs, but oncological outcomes required more evaluation [92,93]. Compared with CRS and HIPEC, PIPAC is more suitable for peritoneal metastases of various origins that cannot be treated by resection. After repeating PIPAC, some cases of unresectable disease could be treated via secondary resection.

There are new methods, such as electrostatic precipitation pressurized intraperitoneal aerosol chemotherapy (ePIPAC), which use electrostatic precipitation of aerosols to achieve stronger penetration and more even distribution [94]. Studies have tested safety and tolerance in treated patients, but efficiency was debatable [95,96]. Another new method, hyperthermic pressurized intraperitoneal aerosol chemotherapy (hPIPAC), which involves the application of cisplatin at temperatures of 38.8–40.2 °C [97], has been proposed and tested recently. Both require further experiments to evaluate feasibility and long-term therapeutic effect.

High-intensity ultrasound (HIUS) has been studied to treat several solid tumors, and the purpose of HIUS was to further enhance tissue penetration, which has been reported [98]. The damage HIUS could cause has also been assessed, and it could yield measurable microscopic changes on the peritoneal surface with minimal damage [99]; however, as a new theory, specifics regarding its usage, safety and combination with other methods, such as CRS plus HIPEC, PIPAC or new biocompatible materials, should be further assessed.

Neoadjuvant intraperitoneal and systemic chemotherapy (NIPS) is a new method aiming to increase possibilities to access CRS, especially for those whose tumor features are not suitable for CRS. A meta-analysis was performed on 8 retrospective studies, including 373 patients with peritoneal metastasis from gastric cancer, 109 of whom continued NIPS treatment because of macroscopic peritoneal metastasis and 265 of whom received surgery for no macroscopic peritoneal metastasis. NIPS combined with surgery significantly improved survival compared to those without surgery, and NIPS could increase the possibility of achieving R0 resection [100]. Other studies supported the idea that NIPS could be used for advanced gastric cancer with peritoneal metastasis [101]. Due to a lack of further clinical data, more clinical trials and research should be conducted to confirm and evaluate this hypothesis.

Drugs targeting adhesion molecules and immunotherapies have shown potential in preventing peritoneal metastasis. Zang et al. found that LPPR4 (which plays a role in promoting peritoneal metastasis of gastric cancer through Sp1/integrin α/FAK signaling) could be a new therapeutic target [102]. The binding of CXCL12 to CXCR4 and CXCR7 on tumor cells leads to antiapoptotic signaling through Bcl-2 and Survivin upregulation; it also promotes EMT through the Rho-ROCK pathway and leads to alterations in cell adhesion molecules. AMD3100 (Plerixafor or Mozobil) is a small molecule CXCR4 antagonist used in clinical trials for gastrointestinal tumors [103] and shows potential prospect. Methods activating immune effects of anti–tumors were investigated due to the high expression of PD-L1 during the process of peritoneal metastasis [104]. CMP-001, a virus-like particle composed of the Qβ bacteriophage capsid protein, encapsulating a CpG-A oligodeoxynucleotide, could activate lasmacytoid dendritic cells and interferon alpha release [105], which might contribute to an anti-tumor response by the development of T-cells [106]. Similarly, oncolytic virotherapy was also classified as another type of immunotherapy; this therapy used viruses as oncolytic vector platforms for the delivery of different treatment agents, such as therapeutic genes, prodrug convertases, toxins, sodium iodide symporter for radiotherapy and immunomodulators [107,108]. JX-594 (pexastimogene devacirepvec, Pexa-vec) is an oncolytic vaccinia virus armed with GM-CSF; a murine version of it shows potential as an anti-tumor by activating dendritic cells and CD8 T cells to enhance their infiltration into peritoneal tumor nodules. Furthermore, it could combine with immune checkpoint inhibitors to induce enhanced immunity to kill metastases [109].

Localized chemotherapy could decrease the toxicity of chemical drugs systemically and maintain a higher concentration in specific areas. In addition to HIPEC and PIPAC, new delivery systems are being studied. Biocompatible carrier systems, such as hydrogels, cells and peptides, have been used for localized drug delivery for the treatment of peritoneal metastasis.

Hydrogels are 3D networks of crosslinked hydrophilic polymer chains that can be formed by different materials and show various abilities. Hydrogels designed for different situations could be sensitive to pH, temperature and physical stimuli, such as light or UV, which means they could protect contents from extreme environments and deliver them in certain areas [110]. Several delivery systems based on hydrogels have shown feasibility in treating peritoneal metastasis (Table 2) [111–114].

Table 2. New delivery systems using hydrogels as a carrier for the treatment of peritoneal carcinomatosis from different origins.

Hydrogels	Drugs	In Vitro	In Vivo	Highlight
linoleic acid-coupled Pluronic F-127 (Plu-CLA) [111]	Docetaxel	Gastric cancer cells TMK1	peritoneal metastasis from gastric cancer	docetaxel–Plu-CLA synergistically inhibits peritoneal metastasis and prolongs survival in a peritoneal gastric cancer model.
Albumin Hydrogel Hybridized with Paclitaxel-Loaded Red Blood Cell Membrane Nanoparticles [112]	Paclitaxel	Gastric cancer cells	peritoneal metastasis from gastric cancer	the hydrogel possesses good tumor growth suppression properties after a single injection.
PTX/PECT (gel) [113]	PTX	Colorectal cancer cells CT-26	peritoneal metastasis from colorectal cancer	sustained drug concentration at peritoneal levels in combination with drug in the form of nanoparticle contributes to the enhanced anti-tumor efficacy.
HA nanogels [114]	Cisplatin	–	peritoneal metastasis from gastric cancer (MKN45P cells)	led to a significantly decreased number of peritoneal nodules, especially those smaller than 1.0 mm.

Another delivery system utilizes cells as carriers. Ling et al. used engineered doxorubicin-loaded M1 macrophages (M1-Dox), which overexpress CCR2 and CCR4, to target cancer cells; M1-Dox transferred drug cargoes into tumor cells via a tunneling nanotube pathway. The results showed that delivering drugs (Dox) from cell to cell was more efficient than lysosomal delivery in terms of effective concentration and drug loading. Furthermore, these cells were not only effective in treating primary tumors, but also had a great advantage in treating metastasis [115]. Functional amyloids produced in bacteria as nanoscale inclusion bodies are a new pathway for treatment. Céspedes et al. used Pseudomonas exotoxin (PE24)-formed bacterial inclusion bodies functionalized with CXCR4 and found that colorectal cancer mouse models treated with these proteins showed significant arrest of tumor growth without toxicity [116]. Albumin, with multiple cellular receptor and ligand binding sites, which are able to bind and transport numerous endogenous and exogenous compounds, could also act as a carrier for chemotherapy drugs targeting peritoneal metastasis, providing a more biocompatible approach for drug delivery [117].

6. Conclusions

Overall, peritoneal metastasis is usually considered a terminal condition in patients and could be derived from several gastrointestinal and gynecological carcinomas. Although an increasing number of molecules have been found to be involved in peritoneal metastasis, the mechanisms of peritoneal metastasis are still complicated, and effective ways to treat them synchronously are lacking. Thus, the specific mechanisms of early tumor cell transfer at the gene and molecular levels should be studied. Recent research on the treatment of peritoneal metastasis has mainly focused on CRS, HIPEC, PIPAC and surgery combined with chemotherapy to local regions. Further studies are needed regarding new methods for enhancing tumor penetration, increasing local drug concentrations, decreasing toxicity and regarding better solutions for patients with advanced peritoneal metastases.

CT is currently the first choice for diagnosis and, combined with MRI or PET/CT, could be more accurate. New materials and methods, such as fluorescence probes, should be proposed for the detection of early minor metastasis so that timely treatment could be taken to prevent further progress.

The tumor microenvironment and interaction between tumor cells and other cells of the peritoneum could be potential targets for treatment. Traditional treatment strategies using chemical drugs need to be improved and new methods need to be created or combined with traditional methods. Furthermore, personalized treatment and health care for patients should also be considered.

Author Contributions: K.R. and X.X. wrote the first draft. T.M., T.S., Y.Z. and H.W. contributed to the critical revision of the manuscript. C.D. and H.Z. reviewed and revised the manuscript. All authors have read and agreed to the published version of the manuscript.

Funding: Supported by the Natural Science Basic Research Program of Shaanxi (Program No. 2019JQ-948).

Institutional Review Board Statement: Not applicable.

Informed Consent Statement: Not applicable.

Conflicts of Interest: The authors declare no conflict of interest.

References

1. Coccolini, F.; Gheza, F.; Lotti, M.; Virzì, S.; Iusco, D.; Ghermandi, C.; Melotti, R.; Baiocchi, G.; Giulini, S.M.; Ansaloni, L.; et al. Peritoneal carcinomatosis. *World J. Gastroenterol. WJG* **2013**, *19*, 6979–6994. [CrossRef]
2. Raptopoulos, V.; Gourtsoyiannis, N. Peritoneal carcinomatosis. *Eur. Radiol.* **2001**, *11*, 2195–2206. [CrossRef]
3. Anwar, A.; Kasi, A. *Peritoneal Cancer*; StatPearls: Tampa, FL, USA, 2020.
4. Quere, P.; Facy, O.; Manfredi, S.; Jooste, V.; Faivre, J.; Lepage, C.; Bouvier, A.-M. Epidemiology, Management, and Survival of Peritoneal Carcinomatosis from Colorectal Cancer: A Population-Based Study. *Dis. Colon Rectum* **2015**, *58*, 743–752. [CrossRef]
5. Feferman, Y.; Solomon, D.; Bhagwandin, S.; Kim, J.; Aycart, S.N.; Feingold, D.; Sarpel, U.; Labow, D.M. Sites of Recurrence After Complete Cytoreduction and Hyperthermic Intraperitoneal Chemotherapy for Patients with Peritoneal Carcinomatosis from Colorectal and Appendiceal Adenocarcinoma: A Tertiary Center Experience. *Ann. Surg. Oncol.* **2019**, *26*, 482–489. [CrossRef]
6. Birgisson, H.; Enblad, M.; Artursson, S.; Ghanipour, L.; Cashin, P.; Graf, W. Patients with colorectal peritoneal metastases and high peritoneal cancer index may benefit from cytoreductive surgery and hyperthermic intraperitoneal chemotherapy. *Eur. J. Surg. Oncol. (EJSO)* **2020**, *46*, 2283–2291. [CrossRef]
7. Deraco, M.; Santoro, N.; Carraro, O.; Inglese, M.G.; Rebuffoni, G.; Guadagni, S.; Somers, D.C.; Vaglini, M. Peritoneal Carcinomatosis: Feature of Dissemination a Review. *Tumori J.* **1999**, *85*, 1–5. [CrossRef]
8. Kastelein, A.W.; Vos, L.M.C.; de Jong, K.H.; van Baal, J.O.A.M.; Nieuwland, R.; van Noorden, C.J.F.; Roovers, J.-P.W.R.; Lok, C.A.R. Embryology, anatomy, physiology and pathophysiology of the peritoneum and the peritoneal vasculature. *Semin. Cell Dev. Biol.* **2018**, *92*, 27–36. [CrossRef]
9. Mutsaers, S.E. Mesothelial cells: Their structure, function and role in serosal repair. *Respirology* **2002**, *7*, 171–191. [CrossRef]
10. Sarfarazi, A.; Lee, G.; Mirjalili, S.A.; Phillips, A.R.; Windsor, J.A.; Trevaskis, N.L. Therapeutic delivery to the peritoneal lymphatics: Current understanding, potential treatment benefits and future prospects. *Int. J. Pharm.* **2019**, *567*, 118456. [CrossRef]
11. Ceelen, W.P.; Bracke, M.E. Peritoneal minimal residual disease in colorectal cancer: Mechanisms, prevention, and treatment. *Lancet Oncol.* **2009**, *10*, 72–79. [CrossRef]
12. Koppe, M.J.; Boerman, O.C.; Oyen, W.J.G.; Bleichrodt, R.P. Peritoneal Carcinomatosis of Colorectal Origin: Incidence and current treatment strategies. *Ann. Surg.* **2006**, *243*, 212–222. [CrossRef]
13. Takebayashi, K.; Murata, S.; Yamamoto, H.; Ishida, M.; Yamaguchi, T.; Kojima, M.; Shimizu, T.; Shiomi, H.; Sonoda, H.; Naka, S.; et al. Surgery-Induced Peritoneal Cancer Cells in Patients Who Have Undergone Curative Gastrectomy for Gastric Cancer. *Ann. Surg. Oncol.* **2014**, *21*, 1991–1997. [CrossRef]
14. Heldin, C.-H.; Rubin, K.; Pietras, K.; Östman, A. High interstitial fluid pressure—An obstacle in cancer therapy. *Nat. Rev. Cancer* **2004**, *4*, 806–813. [CrossRef]
15. Pedrazzani, C.; Kim, H.J.; Park, E.J.; Turri, G.; Zagolin, G.; Foppa, C.; Baik, S.H.; Spolverato, G.; Spinelli, A.; Choi, G.S. Does laparoscopy increase the risk of peritoneal recurrence after resection for pT4 colon cancer? Results of a propensity score-matched analysis from an international cohort. *Eur. J. Surg. Oncol.* **2022**, *48*, 1823–1830. [CrossRef]
16. Du, S.; Miao, J.; Zhu, Z.; Xu, E.; Shi, L.; Ai, S.; Wang, F.; Kang, X.; Chen, H.; Lu, X.; et al. NADPH oxidase 4 regulates anoikis resistance of gastric cancer cells through the generation of reactive oxygen species and the induction of EGFR. *Cell Death Dis.* **2018**, *9*, 948. [CrossRef]
17. Zhang, T.; Wang, B.; Su, F.; Gu, B.; Xiang, L.; Gao, L.; Zheng, P.; Li, X.-M.; Chen, H. TCF7L2 promotes anoikis resistance and metastasis of gastric cancer by transcriptionally activating PLAUR. *Int. J. Biol. Sci.* **2022**, *18*, 4560–4577. [CrossRef]

18. Ye, G.; Yang, Q.; Lei, X.; Zhu, X.; Li, F.; He, J.; Chen, H.; Ling, R.; Zhang, H.; Lin, T.; et al. Nuclear MYH9-induced CTNNB1 transcription, targeted by staurosporin, promotes gastric cancer cell anoikis resistance and metastasis. *Theranostics* **2020**, *10*, 7545–7560. [CrossRef]
19. Dolinschek, R.; Hingerl, J.; Benge, A.; Zafiu, C.; Schüren, E.; Ehmoser, E.K.; Lössner, D.; Reuning, U. Constitutive activation of integrin αvβ3 contributes to anoikis resistance of ovarian cancer cells. *Mol. Oncol.* **2021**, *15*, 503–522. [CrossRef]
20. Shen, W.; Chen, D.; Fu, H.; Liu, S.; Sun, K.; Sun, X. S100A4 protects gastric cancer cells from anoikis through regulation of αv and α5 integrin. *Cancer Sci.* **2011**, *102*, 1014–1018. [CrossRef]
21. Ogishima, J.; Taguchi, A.; Kawata, A.; Kawana, K.; Yoshida, M.; Yoshimatsu, Y.; Sato, M.; Nakamura, H.; Kawata, Y.; Nishijima, A.; et al. The oncogene KRAS promotes cancer cell dissemination by stabilizing spheroid formation via the MEK pathway. *BMC Cancer* **2018**, *18*, 1201. [CrossRef]
22. Yin, M.; Li, X.; Tan, S.; Zhou, H.J.; Ji, W.; Bellone, S.; Xu, X.; Zhang, H.; Santin, A.D.; Lou, G.; et al. Tumor-associated macrophages drive spheroid formation during early transcoelomic metastasis of ovarian cancer. *J. Clin. Investig.* **2016**, *126*, 4157–4173. [CrossRef] [PubMed]
23. Yasumoto, K.; Koizumi, K.; Kawashima, A.; Saitoh, Y.; Arita, Y.; Shinohara, K.; Minami, T.; Nakayama, T.; Sakurai, H.; Takahashi, Y.; et al. Role of the CXCL12/CXCR4 Axis in Peritoneal Carcinomatosis of Gastric Cancer. *Cancer Res.* **2006**, *66*, 2181–2187. [CrossRef] [PubMed]
24. Lv, Z.-D.; Na, D.; Liu, F.-N.; Du, Z.-M.; Sun, Z.; Li, Z.; Ma, X.-Y.; Wang, Z.-N.; Xu, H.-M. Induction of gastric cancer cell adhesion through transforming growth factor-beta1-mediated peritoneal fibrosis. *J. Exp. Clin. Cancer Res.* **2010**, *29*, 139. [CrossRef]
25. Falk, P.; Angenete, E.; Bergström, M.; Ivarsson, M.-L. TGF-β1 promotes transition of mesothelial cells into fibroblast phenotype in response to peritoneal injury in a cell culture model. *Int. J. Surg.* **2013**, *11*, 977–982. [CrossRef] [PubMed]
26. Nishimura, S.; Hirakawa-Chung, K.Y.; Yashiro, M.; Inoue, T.; Matsuoka, T.; Fujihara, T.; Murahashi, K.; Sawada, T.; Nakata, B.; Jikihara, I.; et al. TGF-beta1 produced by gastric cancer cells affects mesothelial cell morphology in peritoneal dissemination. *Int. J. Oncol.* **1998**, *12*, 847–898. [CrossRef]
27. Coppé, J.-P.; Desprez, P.-Y.; Krtolica, A.; Campisi, J. The Senescence-Associated Secretory Phenotype: The Dark Side of Tumor Suppression. *Annu. Rev. Pathol. Mech. Dis.* **2010**, *5*, 99–118. [CrossRef] [PubMed]
28. Fang, Y.; Dou, R.; Huang, S.; Han, L.; Fu, H.; Yang, C.; Song, J.; Zheng, J.; Zhang, X.; Liu, K.; et al. LAMC1-mediated preadipocytes differentiation promoted peritoneum pre-metastatic niche formation and gastric cancer metastasis. *Int. J. Biol. Sci.* **2022**, *18*, 3082–3101. [CrossRef]
29. Xuan, Y.; Wang, H.; Yung, M.M.H.; Chen, F.; Chan, W.-S.; Chan, Y.-S.; Tsui, S.K.W.; Ngan, H.Y.S.; Chan, K.K.L.; Chan, D.W. SCD1/FADS2 fatty acid desaturases equipoise lipid metabolic activity and redox-driven ferroptosis in ascites-derived ovarian cancer cells. *Theranostics* **2022**, *12*, 3534–3552. [CrossRef]
30. Oosterling, S.J.; van der Bij, G.J.; Bögels, M.; van der Sijp, J.R.M.; Beelen, R.H.J.; Meijer, S.; van Egmond, M. Insufficient ability of omental milky spots to prevent peritoneal tumor outgrowth supports omentectomy in minimal residual disease. *Cancer Immunol. Immunother.* **2005**, *55*, 1043–1051. [CrossRef]
31. Miao, Z.-F.; Wang, Z.-N.; Zhao, T.-T.; Xu, Y.-Y.; Gao, J.; Miao, F.; Xu, H.-M. Peritoneal Milky Spots Serve as a Hypoxic Niche and Favor Gastric Cancer Stem/Progenitor Cell Peritoneal Dissemination Through Hypoxia-Inducible Factor 1α. *Stem Cells* **2014**, *32*, 3062–3074. [CrossRef]
32. Cao, L.; Hu, X.; Zhang, J.; Huang, G.; Zhang, Y. The role of the CCL22-CCR4 axis in the metastasis of gastric cancer cells into omental milky spots. *J. Transl. Med.* **2014**, *12*, 267. [CrossRef] [PubMed]
33. Ziprin, P.; Ridgway, P.F.; Pfistermüller, K.L.; Peck, D.H.; Darzi, A.W. ICAM-1 mediated tumor-mesothelial cell adhesion is modulated by IL-6 and TNF-alpha: A potential mechanism by which surgical trauma increases peritoneal metastases. *Cell Commun. Adhes.* **2003**, *10*, 141–154. [CrossRef] [PubMed]
34. Tanaka, H.; Yashiro, M.; Sunami, T.; Ohira, M.; Hirakawa-YS, C.K. Lipid-mediated gene transfection of intercellular adhesion molecule-1 suppresses the peritoneal metastasis of gastric carcinoma. *Int. J. Mol. Med.* **2002**, *10*, 613–617. [CrossRef] [PubMed]
35. Gardner, M.J.; Jones, L.M.; Catterall, J.B.; Turner, G.A. Expression of cell adhesion molecules on ovarian tumour cell lines and mesothelial cells, in relation to ovarian cancer metastasis. *Cancer Lett.* **1995**, *91*, 229–234. [CrossRef]
36. Siyasi, M.; Mahjoubi, F.; Mahjoubi, B.; Shabani, S. Study of VCAM-1 Gene Expression in Normal and Tumoral Tissues in Patients with Colorectal Cancer. *J. Biotechnol. Biomed. Sci.* **2017**, *1*, 19–26. [CrossRef]
37. Arlt, M.J.; Novak-Hofer, I.; Gast, D.; Gschwend, V.; Moldenhauer, G.; Grünberg, J.; Honer, M.; Schubiger, P.A.; Altevogt, P.; Krüger, A. Efficient Inhibition of Intra-Peritoneal Tumor Growth and Dissemination of Human Ovarian Carcinoma Cells in Nude Mice by Anti-L1-Cell Adhesion Molecule Monoclonal Antibody Treatment. *Cancer Res.* **2006**, *66*, 936–943. [CrossRef]
38. Ichikawa, T.; Okugawa, Y.; Toiyama, Y.; Tanaka, K.; Yin, C.; Kitajima, T.; Kondo, S.; Shimura, T.; Ohi, M.; Araki, T.; et al. Clinical significance and biological role of L1 cell adhesion molecule in gastric cancer. *Br. J. Cancer* **2019**, *121*, 1058–1068. [CrossRef]
39. Fournier, G.; Garrido-Urbani, S.; Reymond, N.; Lopez, M. Nectines et nectines-like. *Med. Sci. (Paris)* **2010**, *26*, 273–279. [CrossRef]
40. Bekes, I.; Löb, S.; Holzheu, I.; Janni, W.; Baumann, L.; Wöckel, A.; Wulff, C. Nectin-2 in ovarian cancer: How is it expressed and what might be its functional role? *Cancer Sci.* **2019**, *110*, 1872–1882. [CrossRef]
41. Casey, R.C.; Oegema, T.R., Jr.; Skubitz, K.M.; Pambuccian, S.E.; Grindle, S.M.; Skubitz, A.P.N. Cell membrane glycosylation mediates the adhesion, migration, and invasion of ovarian carcinoma cells. *Clin. Exp. Metastasis* **2003**, *20*, 143–152. [CrossRef]

42. Nakamura, K.; Sawada, K.; Kinose, Y.; Yoshimura, A.; Toda, A.; Nakatsuka, E.; Hashimoto, K.; Mabuchi, S.; Morishige, K.-I.; Kurachi, H.; et al. Exosomes Promote Ovarian Cancer Cell Invasion through Transfer of CD44 to Peritoneal Mesothelial Cells. *Mol. Cancer Res.* **2017**, *15*, 78–92. [CrossRef] [PubMed]
43. Yu, G.; Tang, B.; Yu, P.-W.; Peng, Z.-H.; Qian, F.; Sun, G. Systemic and peritoneal inflammatory response after laparoscopic-assisted gastrectomy and the effect of inflammatory cytokines on adhesion of gastric cancer cells to peritoneal mesothelial cells. *Surg. Endosc.* **2010**, *24*, 2860–2870. [CrossRef]
44. Desgrosellier, J.S.; Cheresh, D.A. Integrins in cancer: Biological implications and therapeutic opportunities. *Nat. Rev. Cancer* **2010**, *10*, 9–22. [CrossRef] [PubMed]
45. Oosterling, S.J.; van der Bij, G.J.; Bögels, M.; Raa, S.T.; Post, J.A.; Meijer, G.A.; Beelen, R.H.; van Egmond, M. Anti-β1 Integrin Antibody Reduces Surgery-Induced Adhesion of Colon Carcinoma Cells to Traumatized Peritoneal Surfaces. *Ann. Surg.* **2008**, *247*, 85–94. [CrossRef] [PubMed]
46. Takatsuki, H.; Komatsu, S.; Sano, R.; Takada, Y.; Tsuji, T. Adhesion of Gastric Carcinoma Cells to Peritoneum Mediated by α3β1 Integrin (VLA-3). *Cancer Res.* **2004**, *64*, 6065–6070. [CrossRef] [PubMed]
47. Scalici, J.M.; Harrer, C.; Allen, A.; Jazaeri, A.; Atkins, K.A.; McLachlan, K.R.; Slack-Davis, J.K. Inhibition of α4β1 integrin increases ovarian cancer response to carboplatin. *Gynecol. Oncol.* **2014**, *132*, 455–461. [CrossRef] [PubMed]
48. Wang, X.; Che, X.; Yu, Y.; Cheng, Y.; Bai, M.; Yang, Z.; Guo, Q.; Xie, X.; Li, D.; Guo, M.; et al. Hypoxia-autophagy axis induces VEGFA by peritoneal mesothelial cells to promote gastric cancer peritoneal metastasis through an integrin α5-fibronectin pathway. *J. Exp. Clin. Cancer Res.* **2020**, *39*, 221. [CrossRef]
49. Lepsenyi, M.; Algethami, N.; Al-Haidari, A.A.; Algaber, A.; Syk, I.; Rahman, M.; Thorlacius, H. CXCL2-CXCR2 axis mediates αV integrin-dependent peritoneal metastasis of colon cancer cells. *Clin. Exp. Metastasis* **2021**, *38*, 401–410. [CrossRef]
50. Asem, M.; Young, A.M.; Oyama, C.; De La Zerda, A.C.; Liu, Y.; Yang, J.; Hilliard, T.S.; Johnson, J.; Harper, E.I.; Guldner, I.; et al. Host Wnt5a Potentiates Microenvironmental Regulation of Ovarian Cancer Metastasis. *Cancer Res.* **2020**, *80*, 1156–1170. [CrossRef]
51. Volz, J.; Köster, S.; Spacek, Z.; Paweletz, N. Characteristic alterations of the peritoneum after carbon dioxide pneumoperitoneum. *Surg. Endosc.* **1999**, *13*, 611–614. [CrossRef]
52. Heath, R.M.; Jayne, D.G.; O'Leary, R.; Morrison, E.E.; Guillou, P.J. Tumour-induced apoptosis in human mesothelial cells: A mechanism of peritoneal invasion by Fas Ligand/Fas interaction. *Br. J. Cancer* **2004**, *90*, 1437–1442. [CrossRef]
53. Yonemura, Y.; Endo, Y.; Fujita, H.; Kimura, K.; Sugiyama, K.; Momiyama, N.; Shimada, H.; Sasaki, T. Inhibition of peritoneal dissemination in human gastric cancer by MMP-7-specific antisense oligonucleotide. *J. Exp. Clin. Cancer Res.* **2001**, *20*, 205–212.
54. Oku, T.; Shimada, K.; Kenmotsu, H.; Ando, Y.; Kurisaka, C.; Sano, R.; Tsuiji, M.; Hasegawa, S.; Fukui, T.; Tsuji, T. Stimulation of Peritoneal Mesothelial Cells to Secrete Matrix Metalloproteinase-9 (MMP-9) by TNF-α: A Role in the Invasion of Gastric Carcinoma Cells. *Int. J. Mol. Sci.* **2018**, *19*, 3961. [CrossRef] [PubMed]
55. Koch, J.; Mönch, D.; Maaß, A.; Mangold, A.; Gužvić, M.; Mürdter, T.; Leibold, T.; Dahlke, M.-H.; Renner, P. Pharmacologic Targeting of MMP2/9 Decreases Peritoneal Metastasis Formation of Colorectal Cancer in a Human Ex Vivo Peritoneum Culture Model. *Cancers* **2022**, *14*, 3760. [CrossRef] [PubMed]
56. Liu, S.; He, J.; Liu, S.; Ji, C.; Guan, W.; Chen, L.; Guan, Y.; Yang, X.; Zhou, Z. Radiomics analysis using contrast-enhanced CT for preoperative prediction of occult peritoneal metastasis in advanced gastric cancer. *Eur. Radiol.* **2020**, *30*, 239–246. [CrossRef]
57. Sun, P.; Li, X.; Wang, L.; Wang, R.; Du, X. Enhanced computed tomography imaging features predict tumor grade in pseudomyxoma peritonei. *Quant. Imaging Med. Surg.* **2022**, *12*, 2321–2331. [CrossRef] [PubMed]
58. Koh, J.-L.; Yan, T.D.; Glenn, D.; Morris, D.L. Evaluation of Preoperative Computed Tomography in Estimating Peritoneal Cancer Index in Colorectal Peritoneal Carcinomatosis. *Ann. Surg. Oncol.* **2009**, *16*, 327–333. [CrossRef]
59. Lim, J.S.; Kim, M.-J.; Yun, M.J.; Oh, Y.T.; Kim, J.H.; Hwang, H.S.; Park, M.-S.; Cha, S.-W.; Lee, J.D.; Noh, S.H.; et al. Comparison of CT and 18F-FDG PET for Detecting Peritoneal Metastasis on the Preoperative Evaluation for Gastric Carcinoma. *Korean J. Radiol.* **2006**, *7*, 249–256. [CrossRef] [PubMed]
60. Esquivel, J.; Chua, T.C. CT versus intraoperative peritoneal cancer index in colorectal cancer peritoneal carcinomatosis: Importance of the difference between statistical significance and clinical relevance. *Ann. Surg. Oncol.* **2009**, *16*, 2662–2663. [CrossRef]
61. Laghi, A.; Bellini, D.; Rengo, M.; Accarpio, F.; Caruso, D.; Biacchi, D.; Di Giorgio, A.; Sammartino, P. Diagnostic performance of computed tomography and magnetic resonance imaging for detecting peritoneal metastases: Systematic review and meta-analysis. *La Radiol. Med.* **2016**, *122*, 1–15. [CrossRef]
62. Sant, I.V.; Engbersen, M.P.; Bhairosing, P.A.; Lambregts, D.M.J.; Beets-Tan, R.G.H.; van Driel, W.J.; Aalbers, A.G.J.; Kok, N.F.M.; Lahaye, M.J. Diagnostic performance of imaging for the detection of peritoneal metastases: A meta-analysis. *Eur. Radiol.* **2020**, *30*, 3101–3112. [CrossRef] [PubMed]
63. Kim, S.-J.; Lee, S.-W. Diagnostic accuracy of ^{18}F-FDG PET/CT for detection of peritoneal carcinomatosis; a systematic review and meta-analysis. *Br. J. Radiol.* **2018**, *91*, 20170519. [CrossRef] [PubMed]
64. Chang, M.-C.; Chen, J.-H.; Liang, J.-A.; Huang, W.-S.; Cheng, K.-Y.; Kao, C.-H. PET or PET/CT for Detection of Peritoneal Carcinomatosis: A Meta-Analysis. *Clin. Nucl. Med.* **2013**, *38*, 623–629. [CrossRef]
65. Sugarbaker, P.H. Peritoneal carcinomatosis of unknown primary site, a study of 25 patients over 30 years. *Eur. J. Surg. Oncol.* **2020**, *46*, 1908–1911. [CrossRef]

66. Nakada, A.; Maruyama, T.; Kamiya, M.; Hanaoka, K.; Urano, Y. Rapid Visualization of Deeply Located Tumors In Vivo by Intravenous Administration of a γ-Glutamyltranspeptidase-Activated Fluorescent Probe. *Bioconjugate Chem.* **2022**, *33*, 523–529. [CrossRef]
67. Llueca, A.; Escrig, J.; Serra-Rubert, A.; Gomez-Quiles, L.; Rivadulla, I.; Játiva-Porcar, R.; Moreno-Clarí, E.; Montañés-Pauls, B.; Granel-Villach, L.; Villegas-Cánovas, C.; et al. Prognostic value of peritoneal cancer index in primary advanced ovarian cancer. *Eur. J. Surg. Oncol.* **2018**, *44*, 163–169. [CrossRef] [PubMed]
68. Bhatt, A.; Yonemura, Y.; Mehta, S.; Benzerdjeb, N.; Kammar, P.; Parikh, L.; Prabhu, A.; Mishra, S.; Shah, M.; Shaikh, S.; et al. The Pathologic Peritoneal Cancer Index (PCI) Strongly Differs from the Surgical PCI in Peritoneal Metastases Arising From Various Primary Tumors. *Ann. Surg. Oncol.* **2020**, *27*, 2985–2996. [CrossRef] [PubMed]
69. Avesani, G.; Arshad, M.; Lu, H.; Fotopoulou, C.; Cannone, F.; Melotti, R.; Aboagye, E.; Rockall, A. Radiological assessment of Peritoneal Cancer Index on preoperative CT in ovarian cancer is related to surgical outcome and survival. *La Radiol. Med.* **2020**, *125*, 770–776. [CrossRef] [PubMed]
70. Evrard, C.; Messina, S.; Sefrioui, D.; Frouin, É.; Auriault, M.-L.; Chautard, R.; Zaanan, A.; Jaffrelot, M.; De La Fouchardière, C.; Aparicio, T.; et al. Heterogeneity of Mismatch Repair Status and Microsatellite Instability between Primary Tumour and Metastasis and Its Implications for Immunotherapy in Colorectal Cancers. *Int. J. Mol. Sci.* **2022**, *23*, 4427. [CrossRef]
71. Bhullar, D.S.; Barriuso, J.; Mullamitha, S.; Saunders, M.P.; O'Dwyer, S.T.; Aziz, O. Biomarker concordance between primary colorectal cancer and its metastases. *EBioMedicine* **2019**, *40*, 363–374. [CrossRef]
72. Ubink, I.; van Eden, W.J.; Snaebjornsson, P.; Kok, N.F.M.; van Kuik, J.; van Grevenstein, W.M.U.; Laclé, M.M.; Sanders, J.; Fijneman, R.J.A.; Elias, S.G.; et al. Histopathological and molecular classification of colorectal cancer and corresponding peritoneal metastases. *Br. J. Surg.* **2018**, *105*, e204–e211. [CrossRef] [PubMed]
73. Fujiyoshi, K.; Yamamoto, G.; Takahashi, A.; Arai, Y.; Yamada, M.; Kakuta, M.; Yamaguchi, K.; Akagi, Y.; Nishimura, Y.; Sakamoto, H.; et al. High concordance rate of KRAS/BRAF mutations and MSI-H between primary colorectal cancer and corresponding metastases. *Oncol. Rep.* **2017**, *37*, 785–792. [CrossRef] [PubMed]
74. Vignot, S.; Lefebvre, C.; Frampton, G.M.; Meurice, G.; Yelensky, R.; Palmer, G.; Capron, F.; Lazar, V.; Hannoun, L.; Miller, V.A.; et al. Comparative analysis of primary tumour and matched metastases in colorectal cancer patients: Evaluation of concordance between genomic and transcriptional profiles. *Eur. J. Cancer* **2015**, *51*, 791–799. [CrossRef] [PubMed]
75. Ariake, K.; Motoi, F.; Ohtsuka, H.; Fukase, K.; Masuda, K.; Mizuma, M.; Hayashi, H.; Nakagawa, K.; Morikawa, T.; Maeda, S.; et al. Predictive risk factors for peritoneal recurrence after pancreatic cancer resection and strategies for its prevention. *Surg. Today* **2017**, *47*, 1434–1442. [CrossRef]
76. Takii, Y.; Mizusawa, J.; Kanemitsu, Y.; Komori, K.; Shiozawa, M.; Ohue, M.; Ikeda, S.; Takiguchi, N.; Kobatake, T.; Ike, H.; et al. The Conventional Technique Versus the No-touch Isolation Technique for Primary Tumor Resection in Patients with Colon Cancer (JCOG1006): A Multicenter, Open-Label, Randomized, Phase III Trial. *Ann. Surg.* **2022**, *275*, 849–855. [CrossRef]
77. Carlier, C.; Mathys, A.; De Jaeghere, E.; Steuperaert, M.; De Wever, O.; Ceelen, W. Tumour tissue transport after intraperitoneal anticancer drug delivery. *Int. J. Hyperth.* **2017**, *33*, 534–542. [CrossRef]
78. Glehen, O.; Kwiatkowski, F.; Sugarbaker, P.H.; Elias, D.; Levine, E.A.; De Simone, M.; Barone, R.; Yonemura, Y.; Cavaliere, F.; Quenet, F.; et al. Cytoreductive Surgery Combined with Perioperative Intraperitoneal Chemotherapy for the Management of Peritoneal Carcinomatosis From Colorectal Cancer: A Multi-Institutional Study. *J. Clin. Oncol.* **2004**, *22*, 3284–3292. [CrossRef]
79. Glehen, O.; Cotte, E.; Schreiber, V.; Sayag-Beaujard, A.C.; Vignal, J.; Gilly, F.N. Intraperitoneal chemohyperthermia and attempted cytoreductive surgery in patients with peritoneal carcinomatosis of colorectal origin. *Br. J. Surg.* **2004**, *91*, 747–754. [CrossRef]
80. Kecmanovic, D.M.; Pavlov, M.J.; Ceranic, M.S.; Sepetkovski, A.V.; Kovacevic, P.A.; Stamenkovic, A.B. Treatment of peritoneal carcinomatosis from colorectal cancer by cytoreductive surgery and hyperthermic perioperative intraperitoneal chemotherapy. *Eur. J. Surg. Oncol. (ESJO)* **2005**, *31*, 147–152. [CrossRef]
81. Rosa, F.; Galiandro, F.; Ricci, R.; Di Miceli, D.; Quero, G.; Fiorillo, C.; Cina, C.; Alfieri, S. Cytoreductive surgery and hyperthermic intraperitoneal chemotherapy (HIPEC) for colorectal peritoneal metastases: Analysis of short- and long-term outcomes. *Langenbeck's Arch. Surg.* **2021**, *406*, 2797–2805. [CrossRef]
82. Quénet, F.; Elias, D.; Roca, L.; Goéré, D.; Ghouti, L.; Pocard, M.; Facy, O.; Arvieux, C.; Lorimier, G.; Pezet, D.; et al. Cytoreductive surgery plus hyperthermic intraperitoneal chemotherapy versus cytoreductive surgery alone for colorectal peritoneal metastases (PRODIGE 7): A multicentre, randomised, open-label, phase 3 trial. *Lancet Oncol.* **2021**, *22*, 256–266. [CrossRef] [PubMed]
83. Van Driel, W.J.; Koole, S.N.; Sikorska, K.; Schagen van Leeuwen, J.H.; Schreuder, H.W.R.; Hermans, R.H.M.; De Hingh, I.H.; Van Der Velden, J.; Arts, H.J.; Massuger, L.F.; et al. Hyperthermic Intraperitoneal Chemotherapy in Ovarian Cancer. *N. Engl. J. Med.* **2018**, *378*, 230–240. [CrossRef] [PubMed]
84. González-Moreno, S.; González-Bayón, L.A.; Ortega-Pérez, G. Hyperthermic intraperitoneal chemotherapy: Rationale and technique. *World J. Gastrointest. Oncol.* **2010**, *2*, 68–75. [CrossRef] [PubMed]
85. De Bree, E.; Michelakis, D.; Stamatiou, D.; Romanos, J.; Zoras, O. Pharmacological principles of intraperitoneal and bidirectional chemotherapy. *Pleura Peritoneum* **2017**, *2*, 47–62. [CrossRef] [PubMed]
86. Valenzuela, C.D.; Levine, E.A.; Mangieri, C.W.; Gawdi, R.; Moaven, O.; Russell, G.; Lundy, M.E.; Perry, K.C.; Votanopoulos, K.I.; Shen, P. Repeat Cytoreductive Surgery with Hyperthermic Intraperitoneal Chemotherapy for Cancers with Peritoneal Metastasis: A 30-year Institutional Experience. *Ann. Surg. Oncol.* **2022**, *29*, 3436–3445. [CrossRef]

87. Moukarzel, L.A.; Ferrando, L.; Dopeso, H.; Stylianou, A.; Basili, T.; Pareja, F.; Paula, A.D.C.; Zoppoli, G.; Abu-Rustum, N.R.; Reis-Filho, J.S.; et al. Hyperthermic intraperitoneal chemotherapy (HIPEC) with carboplatin induces distinct transcriptomic changes in ovarian tumor and normal tissues. *Gynecol. Oncol.* **2022**, *165*, 239–247. [CrossRef]
88. Chia, C.S.; The Big Renape Group; You, B.; Decullier, E.; Vaudoyer, D.; Lorimier, G.; Abboud, K.; Bereder, J.-M.; Arvieux, C.; Boschetti, G.; et al. Patients with Peritoneal Carcinomatosis from Gastric Cancer Treated with Cytoreductive Surgery and Hyperthermic Intraperitoneal Chemotherapy: Is Cure a Possibility? *Ann. Surg. Oncol.* **2016**, *23*, 1971–1979. [CrossRef]
89. Nadiradze, G.; Horvath, P.; Sautkin, Y.; Archid, R.; Weinreich, F.-J.; Königsrainer, A.; Reymond, M.A. Overcoming Drug Resistance by Taking Advantage of Physical Principles: Pressurized Intraperitoneal Aerosol Chemotherapy (PIPAC). *Cancers* **2019**, *12*, 34. [CrossRef]
90. Kepenekian, V.; Péron, J.; You, B.; Bonnefoy, I.; Villeneuve, L.; Alyami, M.; Bakrin, N.; Rousset, P.; Benzerdjeb, N.; Glehen, O. Non-resectable Malignant Peritoneal Mesothelioma Treated with Pressurized Intraperitoneal Aerosol Chemotherapy (PIPAC) Plus Systemic Chemotherapy Could Lead to Secondary Complete Cytoreductive Surgery: A Cohort Study. *Ann. Surg. Oncol.* **2021**, *29*, 2104–2113. [CrossRef]
91. Alyami, M.; Mercier, F.; Siebert, M.; Bonnot, P.-E.; Laplace, N.; Villeneuve, L.; Passot, G.; Glehen, O.; Bakrin, N.; Kepenekian, V. Unresectable peritoneal metastasis treated by pressurized intraperitoneal aerosol chemotherapy (PIPAC) leading to cytoreductive surgery and hyperthermic intraperitoneal chemotherapy. *Eur. J. Surg. Oncol.* **2021**, *47*, 128–133. [CrossRef]
92. Taibi, A.; Sgarbura, O.; Hübner, M.; Bardet, S.M.; Alyami, M.; Bakrin, N.; Fontanier, S.D.; Eveno, C.; Gagniere, J.; Pache, B.; et al. Feasibility and Safety of Oxaliplatin-Based Pressurized Intraperitoneal Aerosol Chemotherapy with or without Intraoperative Intravenous 5-Fluorouracil and Leucovorin for Colorectal Peritoneal Metastases: A Multicenter Comparative Cohort Study. *Ann. Surg. Oncol.* **2022**, *29*, 5243–5251. [CrossRef] [PubMed]
93. Rovers, K.P.; Wassenaar, E.C.E.; Lurvink, R.J.; Creemers, G.-J.M.; Burger, J.W.A.; Los, M.; Huysentruyt, C.J.R.; van Lijnschoten, G.; Nederend, J.; Lahaye, M.J.; et al. Pressurized Intraperitoneal Aerosol Chemotherapy (Oxaliplatin) for Unresectable Colorectal Peritoneal Metastases: A Multicenter, Single-Arm, Phase II Trial (CRC-PIPAC). *Ann. Surg. Oncol.* **2021**, *28*, 5311–5326. [CrossRef] [PubMed]
94. Kakchekeeva, T.; Demtröder, C.; Herath, N.I.; Griffiths, D.; Torkington, J.; Solaß, W.; Dutreix, M.; Reymond, M.A. In Vivo Feasibility of Electrostatic Precipitation as an Adjunct to Pressurized Intraperitoneal Aerosol Chemotherapy (ePIPAC). *Ann. Surg. Oncol.* **2016**, *23*, 592–598. [CrossRef] [PubMed]
95. Taibi, A.; Farinha, H.T.; Fontanier, S.D.; Sayedalamin, Z.; Hübner, M.; Sgarbura, O. Pressurized Intraperitoneal Aerosol Chemotherapy Enhanced by Electrostatic Precipitation (ePIPAC) for Patients with Peritoneal Metastases. *Ann. Surg. Oncol.* **2021**, *28*, 3852–3860. [CrossRef] [PubMed]
96. Graversen, M.; Detlefsen, S.; Ellebaek, S.B.; Fristrup, C.W.; Pfeiffer, P.; Mortensen, M.B. Pressurized IntraPeritoneal Aerosol Chemotherapy with one minute of electrostatic precipitation (ePIPAC) is feasible, but the histological tumor response in peritoneal metastasis is insufficient. *Eur. J. Surg. Oncol.* **2020**, *46*, 155–159. [CrossRef]
97. Bachmann, C.; Sautkin, I.; Nadiradze, G.; Archid, R.; Weinreich, F.J.; Königsrainer, A.; Reymond, M.A. Technology development of hyperthermic pressurized intraperitoneal aerosol chemotherapy (hPIPAC). *Surg. Endosc.* **2021**, *35*, 6358–6365. [CrossRef]
98. Mikolajczyk, A.; Khosrawipour, T.; Martino, A.; Kulas, J.; Pieczka, M.; Zacharski, M.; Nicpon, J.; Khosrawipour, V. Enabling Microparticle Imprinting to Achieve Penetration and Local Endurance in the Peritoneum via High-Intensity Ultrasound (HIUS) for the Treatment of Peritoneal Metastasis. *Int. J. Surg. Oncol.* **2020**, *2020*, 9679385. [CrossRef]
99. Lau, H.; Khosrawipour, T.; Mikolajczyk, A.; Frelkiewicz, P.; Nicpon, J.; Arafkas, M.; Pigazzi, A.; Knoefel, W.T.; Khosrawipour, V. Intraperitoneal chemotherapy of the peritoneal surface using high-intensity ultrasound (HIUS): Investigation of technical feasibility, safety and possible limitations. *J. Cancer* **2020**, *11*, 7209–7215. [CrossRef]
100. Gong, Y.; Wang, P.; Zhu, Z.; Zhang, J.; Huang, J.; Wang, T.; Chen, J.; Xu, H. Benefits of Surgery After Neoadjuvant Intraperitoneal and Systemic Chemotherapy for Gastric Cancer Patients with Peritoneal Metastasis: A Meta-Analysis. *J. Surg. Res.* **2020**, *245*, 234–243. [CrossRef]
101. Fujiwara, Y.; Takiguchi, S.; Nakajima, K.; Miyata, H.; Yamasaki, M.; Kurokawa, Y.; Okada, K.; Mori, M.; Doki, Y. Neoadjuvant Intraperitoneal and Systemic Chemotherapy for Gastric Cancer Patients with Peritoneal Dissemination. *Ann. Surg. Oncol.* **2011**, *18*, 3726–3731. [CrossRef]
102. Zang, D.; Zhang, C.; Li, C.; Fan, Y.; Li, Z.; Hou, K.; Che, X.; Liu, Y.; Qu, X. LPPR4 promotes peritoneal metastasis via Sp1/integrin α/FAK signaling in gastric cancer. *Am. J. Cancer Res.* **2020**, *10*, 1026–1044. [PubMed]
103. Daniel, S.K.; Seo, Y.D.; Pillarisetty, V.G. The CXCL12-CXCR4/CXCR7 axis as a mechanism of immune resistance in gastrointestinal malignancies. *Semin. Cancer Biol.* **2020**, *65*, 176–188. [CrossRef] [PubMed]
104. Abiko, K.; Mandai, M.; Hamanishi, J.; Yoshioka, Y.; Matsumura, N.; Baba, T.; Yamaguchi, K.; Murakami, R.; Yamamoto, A.; Kharma, B.; et al. PD-L1 on Tumor Cells Is Induced in Ascites and Promotes Peritoneal Dissemination of Ovarian Cancer through CTL Dysfunction. *Clin. Cancer Res.* **2013**, *19*, 1363–1374. [CrossRef] [PubMed]
105. Miller, A.M.; Lemke-Miltner, C.D.; Blackwell, S.; Tomanek-Chalkley, A.; Gibson-Corely, K.N.; Coleman, K.L.; Weiner, G.J.; Chan, C.H.F. Intraperitoneal CMP-001: A Novel Immunotherapy for Treating Peritoneal Carcinomatosis of Gastrointestinal and Pancreaticobiliary Cancer. *Ann. Surg. Oncol.* **2021**, *28*, 1187–1197. [CrossRef]
106. Sabree, S.A.; Voigt, A.P.; Blackwell, S.E.; Vishwakarma, A.; Chimenti, M.S.; Salem, A.K.; Weiner, G.J. Direct and indirect immune effects of CMP-001, a virus-like particle containing a TLR9 agonist. *J. Immunother. Cancer* **2021**, *9*, e002484. [CrossRef]

107. Engeland, C.E.; Bell, J.C. Introduction to Oncolytic Virotherapy. In *Oncolytic Viruses*; Methods in Molecular Biology; Humana: New York, NY, USA, 2020; Volume 2058, pp. 1–6. [CrossRef]
108. Twumasi-Boateng, K.; Pettigrew, J.L.; Kwok, Y.Y.E.; Bell, J.C.; Nelson, B.H. Oncolytic viruses as engineering platforms for combination immunotherapy. *Nat. Rev. Cancer* **2018**, *18*, 419–432. [CrossRef]
109. Lee, Y.S.; Lee, W.S.; Kim, C.W.; Lee, S.J.; Yang, H.; Kong, S.J.; Ning, J.; Yang, K.-M.; Kang, B.; Kim, W.R.; et al. Oncolytic vaccinia virus reinvigorates peritoneal immunity and cooperates with immune checkpoint inhibitor to suppress peritoneal carcinomatosis in colon cancer. *J. Immunother. Cancer* **2020**, *8*, e000857. [CrossRef]
110. Norouzi, M.; Nazari, B.; Miller, D.W. Injectable hydrogel-based drug delivery systems for local cancer therapy. *Drug Discov. Today* **2016**, *21*, 1835–1849. [CrossRef]
111. Bae, W.K.; Park, M.S.; Lee, J.H.; Hwang, J.E.; Shim, H.J.; Cho, S.H.; Kim, D.-E.; Ko, H.M.; Cho, C.-S.; Park, I.-K.; et al. Docetaxel-loaded thermoresponsive conjugated linoleic acid-incorporated poloxamer hydrogel for the suppression of peritoneal metastasis of gastric cancer. *Biomaterials* **2013**, *34*, 1433–1441. [CrossRef]
112. Qian, H.; Qian, K.; Cai, J.; Yang, Y.; Zhu, L.; Liu, B. Therapy for Gastric Cancer with Peritoneal Metastasis Using Injectable Albumin Hydrogel Hybridized with Paclitaxel-Loaded Red Blood Cell Membrane Nanoparticles. *ACS Biomater. Sci. Eng.* **2019**, *5*, 1100–1112. [CrossRef]
113. Xu, S.; Fan, H.; Yin, L.; Zhang, J.; Dong, A.; Deng, L.; Tang, H. Thermosensitive hydrogel system assembled by PTX-loaded copolymer nanoparticles for sustained intraperitoneal chemotherapy of peritoneal carcinomatosis. *Eur. J. Pharm. Biopharm.* **2016**, *104*, 251–259. [CrossRef] [PubMed]
114. Ohta, S.; Hiramoto, S.; Amano, Y.; Emoto, S.; Yamaguchi, H.; Ishigami, H.; Kitayama, J.; Ito, T. Intraperitoneal Delivery of Cisplatin via a Hyaluronan-Based Nanogel/in Situ Cross-Linkable Hydrogel Hybrid System for Peritoneal Dissemination of Gastric Cancer. *Mol. Pharm.* **2017**, *14*, 3105–3113. [CrossRef] [PubMed]
115. Guo, L.; Zhang, Y.; Yang, Z.; Peng, H.; Wei, R.; Wang, C.; Feng, M. Tunneling Nanotubular Expressways for Ultrafast and Accurate M1 Macrophage Delivery of Anticancer Drugs to Metastatic Ovarian Carcinoma. *ACS Nano* **2019**, *13*, 1078–1096. [CrossRef] [PubMed]
116. Céspedes, M.V.; Cano-Garrido, O.; Álamo, P.; Sala, R.; Gallardo, A.; Serna, N.; Falgàs, A.; Voltà-Durán, E.; Casanova, I.; Sánchez-Chardi, A.; et al. Engineering Secretory Amyloids for Remote and Highly Selective Destruction of Metastatic Foci. *Adv. Mater.* **2020**, *32*, e1907348. [CrossRef]
117. Van De Sande, L.; Cosyns, S.; Willaert, W.; Ceelen, W. Albumin-based cancer therapeutics for intraperitoneal drug delivery: A review. *Drug Deliv.* **2020**, *27*, 40–53. [CrossRef]

Journal of
Clinical Medicine

MDPI

Article

Peritoneal Mesothelioma in a High Volume Peritoneal Surface Malignancies Unit

Fernando Pereira [1,2,*], Mónica Pereira [2], Israel Manzanedo [1,2], Ángel Serrano [1,2] and Estibalitz Pérez-Viejo [1,2]

1 Peritoneal Surface Malignancies Unit, Department of Surgery, Hospital Universitario de Fuenlabrada, 28942 Madrid, Spain
2 Faculty of Health Sciences, School of Medicine, Universidad Rey Juan Carlos, 28933 Madrid, Spain
* Correspondence: fernando.pereira@salud.madrid.org; Tel.: +34-16006455

Abstract: Diffuse malignant peritoneal mesothelioma (PM) is a rare neoplasm, traditionally associated with a poor prognosis. There are other varieties of PM that are even less frequent and of uncertain malignancy. Cytoreductive surgery (CRS) with hyperthermic intraperitoneal chemotherapy (HIPEC) has achieved prolonged survival in selected patients. The aim of this study is to analyze the patients with PM assessed in our center. Clinicopathological characteristics, diagnostic procedures and survival results from patients with PM appraised at our unit, according to the applied treatment, were analyzed. Seventeen patients were assessed between 2007 and 2019. Three cases had multicystic PM that were treated with complete CRS + HIPEC; all patients are alive and free of disease after a long follow-up. Three other cases had biphasic PM; a curative treatment could be performed in none of them, and their survival was minimal (<6 moths). Lastly, 11 cases with epithelioid PM were treated. Two cases were considered unresectable at laparoscopy (PCI 39); one of them had a long survival (67 months) with three iterative laparoscopic palliatives HIPECs for refractory ascites. The other nine cases were treated with curative CRS + HIPEC, with a median PCI of 14 (range 4–25), and a median overall survival (OS) of 58 months, with a 5-year OS of 47.4%. In conclusion, CRS + HIPEC, when possible, appears to be the optimal treatment for patients with PM. Knowledge of this therapeutic option is crucial, both to offer it to patients and to avoid delays in their referral to appropriate centers for treatment.

Keywords: peritoneal mesothelioma; epithelioid subtype; cytoreductive surgery; HIPEC

1. Introduction

Diffuse malignant peritoneal mesothelioma (DMPM) is an aggressive neoplasm arising from mesothelial cells of the peritoneal serosa, and may affect the peritoneal surface more or less extensively. The incidence of DMPM is very low (0.2–3 cases/million inhabitants/year) [1], much lower than that of pleural mesothelioma [2], and less related to asbestos exposure than the pleural variety [1]. The most common histological subtype is epithelioid (75% of cases), followed by sarcomatoid (13%) and biphasic (6%) [3]. Traditional treatment of DMPM is systemic chemotherapy (CT) with palliative surgery on demand, resulting in a fatal prognosis. The median overall survival (OS) with contemporary systemic CT (pemetrexed + platinum) [4] is about 12 months, with response rates around 30%. The implementation of cytoreductive surgery (CRS) with hypertermic intraperitoneal chemotherapy (HIPEC), especially in the last two decades, has been a therapeutic milestone, reaching survival rates of 53 months (range 34–92 months) with a 5-year OS of 47% [5]. Nowadays, it is considered the treatment of choice for all those patients in whom complete cytoreduction seems possible. Careful patient selection and center experience are essential to optimize both postoperative and long-term survival outcomes [6,7]. HIPEC has also been successfully used as a palliative treatment for refractory ascites in patients with unresectable disease [8,9].

There are two other varieties of diffuse peritoneal mesothelioma (PM) that are considered borderline (well-differentiated papillary and multicystic), as they can relapse after surgery and exceptionally progress to DMPM [10,11]. In these varieties, CRS + HIPEC is considered a better alternative than isolated CRS [7].

Due to the low incidence of the disease, there are very few centers with large series of PM treated with CRS + HIPEC [12,13]. In Spain, we have only found a small series (7 patients) published in 2007 [14]. However, two essential multi-center studies [5,15], a meta-analysis [16] and multiple reviews have been published, among which it should be highlighted the recent PSOGI/EURACAN guideline [7].

The aim of this study is to analyze the outcome of patients with PM assessed at our high volume Peritoneal Surface Malignancies Unit (in which we perform around 100 annual CRS + HIPEC procedures for different indications, including PM).

2. Materials and Methods

Patients with PM referred to our Peritoneal Surface Malignancy Unit for diagnostic and/or therapeutic evaluation were analyzed. Treatment options were evaluated in the Multidisciplinary Tumor Board (MTB), taking into account the performance status, the histological variety and the extent of the disease in imaging test or by laparoscopy, including the indication of preoperative CT (pemetrexed-platinum) in potentially resectable cases with malignant varieties.

Patients for whom surgery was considered to be beneficial were operated with initial curative intention, although the final decision on cytoreduction was made during the intervention, after a precise assessment of the extent of the disease. CRS was performed with a variety of selective peritonectomies and visceral resections, and it was at least attempted that residual disease remain millimetric in those cases in which complete cytoreduction was not possible. In patients in whom significant cytoreduction was achieved (CCS 0-1), HIPEC with Cisplatin 100 mg/m^2 + Doxorubicin 15 mg/m^2 was carried out for 90 min. In two of these patients, during the early years of our program, EPIC (early postoperative intraperitoneal chemotherapy) was also used during the first 3–5th postoperative days (with paclitaxel 20 mg/m^2 in 1000 cc of peritofundin). Finally, in cases where the disease was considered unresectable, palliative HIPEC was carried out (laparoscopically when possible) in those with malignant ascites.

Major postoperative complications were recorded (Dindo–Clavien classification [17]). Patients were reevaluated again by the MTB after discharge, and a final decision was made on the need of postoperative CT and the follow-up protocol. In case of recurrence, patients were treated according to a new decision of the MTB, even with surgery (including the possibility of additional CRS + HIPEC) when the appropriate criteria were met.

Informed consent was obtained from all individuals included in this study. The research has been approved by the authors' institutional review board.

Statistical study: Qualitative variables are described with their distribution frequencies. Quantitative variables are described with their medians and ranges. The Kaplan–Meier method was used for survival analysis. All statistical analyses were performed using SPSS 25.0.

3. Results

From 2007 to 2019, 17 patients with PM were assessed in our Peritoneal Surface Malignancies Unit. Data were analyzed in February 2020. The clinical characteristics are summarized in Table 1. Only five patients were initially evaluated in our own center, while the rest came from other centers in Madrid ($n = 7$) or other regions of Spain ($n = 5$).

Table 1. Descriptive statistics.

	Multicystic	Biphasic	Epithelioid
N° of patients	3	3	11
Origin: our center/other centers	1/2	2/1	2/9
Age (median)	51	64	57
Sex (female/male)	3/0	1/2	5/6
Asbestos exposure	0	0	1
Previous abdominal surgeries	1	0	1
Unresectable	0	3	2

Three of the cases were women with multicystic PM, all initially asymptomatic and discovered incidentally at gynecological examinations. In one of them, two previous incomplete cytoreductions had been performed in another center. All three were treated with complete CRS (CCS 0) + HIPEC, with a median PCI (Peritoneal Cancer Index) of 18 (range 8–21). None had serious complications (only one had a minor complication consisting of low-grade fever with no clear focus), and the median hospital stay was 7 days (range 7–13). After a median follow-up of 59 months (range 33–127), all remain alive and free of disease.

Three other cases correspond to biphasic DMPM. One 83-year-old patient was diagnosed at an urgent and palliative surgery for bowel obstruction, with post-operative death after 5 days. The other two patients presented with progressive abdominal distension and constitutional syndrome. One of them was admitted to our center for study and a laparoscopy was performed, declaring the tumor unresectable (PCI 30). The last patient was diagnosed (by laparoscopy) and received CT (pemetrexed + cisplatin) in other hospital; in our center, a second restaging laparoscopy was performed and an attempt of CRS + HIPEC was made, but it was considered finally unresectable (PCI 39), performing a palliative HIPEC for malignant ascites. Both patients received palliative CT but had minimal survival (6 months).

Finally, 11 cases with epithelioid DMPM have been treated. All debuted with variable patterns of distension and/or abdominal pain and/or constitutional syndrome, except for one asymptomatic case diagnosed after the removal of an umbilical nodule (suspected umbilical hernia).

In two finally unresectable cases (both women), the diagnosis of extensive disease was made at an initial laparoscopy, followed by neoadjuvant CT (NACT), both being definitely unresectable (PCI 39) after a second restaging laparoscopy. In one of them, palliative HIPEC was applied (in the 2nd laparoscopy) for the treatment of ascites. This patient (in whom laparoscopic HIPEC was subsequently repeated twice for refractory ascites) had a long survival (67 months). The other patient was lost after 4 months of follow-up (she came from outside Madrid).

In the other nine cases of epithelioid DMPM, CRS + HIPEC was performed with curative intent (CCS 0 in 7, CCS 1 in 2). In 7/9, a previous staging laparoscopy had been performed and five of them received NACT for extensive disease. In addition, the remaining two patients who did not undergo staging laparoscopy had also received NACT previously in other hospitals (a total of seven patients with NACT) and they were referred to our center after confirming response (in one) or stable disease (in the other), being then operated without previous laparoscopy, both with low PCI (6 and 4) at surgery. Median surgical PCI in the nine patients was 14 (range 4–25) with the following distribution: PCI < 10 in 3 cases, PCI 10–20 in three cases, and PCI > 20 in three cases. The peritoneal/visceral resection procedures are detailed in Table 2.

Table 2. Resections performed in epithelioid PM cases with complete cytoreduction ($n = 9$).

Procedures	Number
Major omentectomy	9
Appendectomy	7
Right diaphragm peritonectomy	6
Left diaphragm peritonectomy	4
Morrison peritonectomy	4
Hepatoduodenal ligament	4
Lateral parietal peritonectomy	4
Pelvic peritonectomy	4
Cholecystectomy	4
Splenectomy	3
Anterior parietal peritonectomy	3
Right hemicolectomy	3
Total hysterectomy	1
Bilateral salpingo—oophorectomy	1
Anterior resection of rectum	1
Superior recess of the omental bursa	1
Hepatic capsulectomy (partial)	1
Small bowel resection	1
Electrofulgurations *	5

* mesenteric or left diaphragm.

The median duration of the nine CRS + HIPEC procedures was 360 min (range 300–510). Two patients also received EPIC. One patient died on the 11th postoperative day after extensive (PCI 25) and complete cytoreduction (CCS 0) with politransfusion, due to multiorgan failure secondary to systemic inflammatory response syndrome and sepsis, without surgical complications. Only one other patient had serious complications (grade III Dindo-Clavien) with organ-space SSI and reoperation for intestinal leak and evisceration. The rate of severe complications was 22.2% (2/9), including the exitus. Another four patients had minor complications (acute urinary retention, ileus, urinary tract infection, seroma), with a total of complications of any grade of 66.6% (6/9). The median hospital stay was 11 days (range 6–30).

Adjuvant CT was administered in four of the seven patients who had received NACT, all after extensive cytoreductions (PCI > 13). Two patients who received NACT but had low surgical PCI (6 and 4) did not receive adjuvant CT. Only one patient with high PCI (16), who had received NACT, did not receive postoperative CT due to poor postoperative performance status.

Of the eight patients in whom CRS was possible with curative intent and who survived the intervention (excluding the postoperative exitus), five have relapsed (four in the peritoneum and one axillary lymph node recurrence). Surgical rescue was attempted in all five, but 3/4 peritoneal recurrences were considered unresectable at re-laparotomy (in one patient on two occasions); the planned HIPEC was also ruled out in two of them (twice in one of these patients) and two palliative HIPECs were performed in the third (with ascites and imprecise PCI for encapsulating peritoneal sclerosis), who is still alive despite persistent disease 110 months after the first surgery (very prolonged OS). In the other two relapses (one peritoneal and the other axillary lymphatic), complete resection was achieved without subsequent recurrence (with CRS + HIPEC in the first and bilateral axillary lymphadenectomy in the latter, although this one has died in the follow-up due to another cause) (Figure 1).

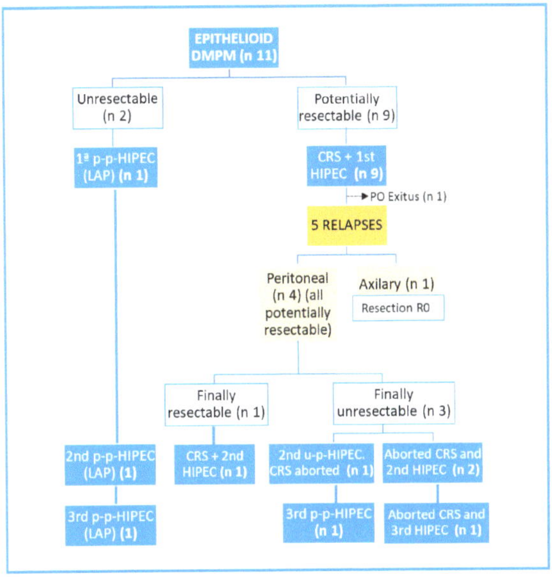

Figure 1. Flowchart of programmed, performed, palliative/curative and aborted HIPECs in epithelioid DMPM. "DMPM": diffuse malignant peritoneal mesothelioma; "CRS": cytoreductive surgery; "p-p−HIPEC": planned-palliative HIPEC; "u-p−HIPEC": unplanned-palliative HIPEC; "LAP": laparoscopic; "PO Exitus": postoperative exitus.

Perioperative data of all CRS + HIPEC performed with curative intention, three in multicystic PM and ten in epithelioid DMPM (9 at initial presentation and 1 at relapse) are summarized in Table 3.

Table 3. Perioperative data of all curative CRS + HIPEC for peritoneal mesothelioma.

	Multicystic (n = 3)	**Epithelioid (n = 10)**	**Total (n = 13)**
Staging laparoscopy	0	7	*
Neoadj treatment	NA	7	*
surgical PCI, median (range)	18 (8–21)	14 (4–25)	15 (4–25)
Duration (min), median (range)	350 (240–350)	360 (300–510)	360 (240–510)
Transfusion	0	1	1
Complic grade ≥ III	0	2	2 (15.3%)
Complic any grade	1	6	7 (53.8%)
Reoperation	0	1	1
Mortality	0	1	1 (7.6%)
Length of stay (days), median (range)	7 (7–13)	11 (6–30)	10 (6–30)
Adjuvant treatment	NA	4	*

"NA": not applicable. * Not recorded since, in multicystic PM, there is no indication for systemic chemotherapy.

With a median follow-up of 49 months, the median OS in the nine patients with epithelioid DMPM in whom CRS with curative intent was possible (including the postoperative exitus) is 58 months, with a 5-year OS of 47.4%. The median disease-free survival (DFS) is 17 months, with a 4-year DFS of 38% (Figure 2).

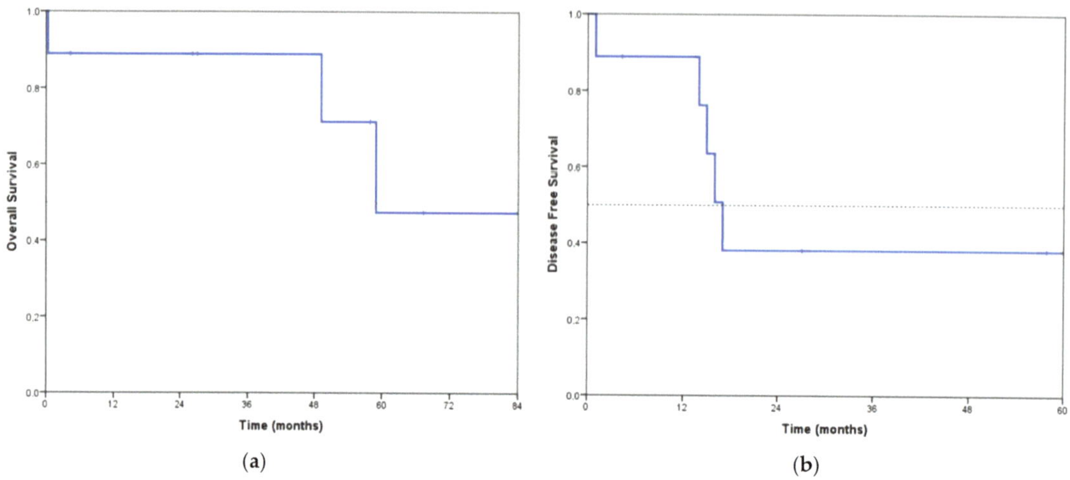

Figure 2. Overall survival (**a**) and disease−free survival (**b**) in the nine epithelioid peritoneal mesotheliomas with complete CRS + HIPEC.

In total, we programmed 22 HIPECs in 14 patients, four of which had initial planned-palliative intention (one first, one second and two third HIPECs). Finally, of the 18 attempts of CRS + HIPEC with curative intent (13 in first attempt, 4 in second attempt and 1 in third attempt) only 13 were curative (12/13 in first attempt, 1/4 in second attempt and 0/1 in 3rd attempt). Therefore, CRS was aborted in 5/18 (27.7%) attempts of CRS + HIPEC with curative intent, and the number of palliative HIPECs increased from 4 to 6 (as an unplanned-palliative HIPEC was performed in 2 of these 5 aborted-CRS cases). In summary, we finally performed a total of 19 HIPECs (6 palliative and 13 with curative intent). The six palliative HIPECs have been performed in three patients, and three of them have been carried out by laparoscopy (all in the same patient).

A total of 18 of the 22 scheduled HIPECs were planned in 10 epithelioid DMPM (Figure 1), 4 of which had initial planned-palliative intention (one first, one second and two third HIPECs). Finally, of the 14 attempts of CRS + HIPEC with curative intent (9 in first attempt, 4 in second attempt and 1 in third attempt), only 10 were curative (9/9 in first attempt, 1/4 in second attempt and 0/1 in 3rd attempt). Therefore, CRS was aborted in 4/14 (28.5%) attempts of CRS + HIPEC with curative intent in epithelioid DMPM, and the number of palliative HIPECs in epithelioid DMPM increased from 4 to 5 (as it was performed a 2nd unplanned-palliative HIPEC in 1 of the 3 aborted-CRS cases with finally unresectable peritoneal relapse).

4. Discussion

Due to the low incidence of PM, it is of utmost importance to concentrate patients in centers with expertise in the treatment of peritoneal diseases, in which the learning curve (both in the selection of patients and in the highly complex surgical procedures) no longer has a negative impact on the outcomes. Of the seventeen patients with PM assessed at our center, only five were initially evaluated in our own hospital, while the rest were referred from other centers.

Precise patient selection for CRS + HIPEC is crucial in DMPM to avoid unnecessary laparotomies and save surgical resources. Thus, it is highly recommended to use laparoscopic staging whenever possible [18], even though there still is a risk of underestimating the real extension of the disease [19]. In our patients, staging laparoscopy was performed on 2/3 patients with biphasic PM (not on the one diagnosed in urgent surgery for bowel obstruction), and on 9/11 patients with epithelioid PM. In some patients (one biphasic and two epithelioid), even two laparoscopies were carried out, one diagnostic of the unresectable mesothelioma and another one after neoadjuvant chemotherapy (NACT) to reevaluate a chance of cytoreduction.

Initial laparoscopies allowed the exclusion of three patients for CRS (in one of them palliative laparoscopic HIPEC was performed), and of the first 13 surgeries scheduled with a curative intent, only one was suspended (a biphasic PM in which there seemed to be a possibility of cytoreduction at laparoscopy after NACT, but a palliative HIPEC was finally performed). However, of the five curative-intent surgeries scheduled for relapses (4 in second and 1 in third attempts), four CRS had to be discarded due to intraoperative irresectability (one with palliative HIPEC). In these cases, the role of laparoscopic assessment is very limited (or impossible) due to previous extensive open surgery, and there is no alternative but to estimate the possibility of cytoreduction based on imaging tests. Overall, 5 of the 18 attempts of CRS + HIPEC with a curative intent were aborted (38.4%), a result that is consistent with the rate of incomplete CRS reported in the literature (33%, range 7–57%) [16].

CRS + HIPEC procedures in specialized centers are associated with a mortality rate of 0.9–5.8% and serious perioperative morbidity of 12–52% [20]. In our PM series, there was one post-operative exitus among the 13 CRS + HIPEC procedures. This mortality is high (1/13 = 7.6%), but no conclusions can be drawn from such a small series. In our overall series of CRS + HIPEC for any indication (including colon, gastric, ovarian cancer, peritoneal pseudomyxoma, PM and non-conventional indications), currently exceeding 900 cases, postoperative mortality is 3%, similar to that of most expert centers. However, serious morbidity (Dindo-Clavien III–V, including the postoperative exitus) of this series is low, only present in 2 of the 13 procedures (15.3%) (Table 3).

Different cytotoxic drugs have been used for HIPEC in PM, mainly cisplatin and mitomycin C, administered alone or in combination with doxorubicin or other drugs. It seems that the best result is obtained with combined schemes [21], based on platinum at least when CRS is complete [15].

The use of NACT in DMPM is under debate, and there are even authors who consider it harmful when a complete CRS can be achieved [22,23]. It is usually administered when there are doubts about resectability. In our series, 7/9 patients with epithelioid DMPM treated with complete CRS + HIPEC had received NACT with pemetrexed-cisplatin. The recent international recommendations of PSOGI/EURACAN specify three scenarios: (1) resectable patients, (2) clearly unresectable patients, and (3) borderline resectable patients [7]. Primary CRS + HIPEC is considered the treatment of choice when the disease is resectable. In patients with unresectable or borderline disease, there is the option of neoadjuvant CT (even bidirectional with intraperitoneal pemetrexed + intravenous cisplatin), having reported surgical rescues in up to 50% of cases [24]. In this regard (conversion to resectability), great expectations have recently been raised with the use of PIPAC (pressurized intraperitoneal aerosol chemotherapy) in different indications [25], and a specific trial in DMPM has even been designed [26].

The use of adjuvant CT after CRS + HIPEC is considered beneficial, especially in the presence of any adverse prognostic factor (CCS $\geq$ 1, sarcomatoid or biphasic subtypes, lymph node metastases, high PCI or Ki-67 > 9%) [7]. Nevertheless, adjuvant CT can be avoided in patients with favorable prognosis. In our series, five of the nine patients with epithelioid PM treated with complete CRS + HIPEC did not receive postoperative CT. However, this includes two cases that would have been candidates but did not receive it for other reasons: the postoperative exitus and another patient with poor postoperative performance status.

Only a few multi-institutional registries have managed to gather a large number of patients with PM treated with CRS + HIPEC. The best known are those published by Yan et al. in 2009 [5] (405 patients with a median OS of 53 months and 5-year OS of 47%) and Alexander et al. in 2013 (211 patients from three US institutions with a median OS of 38.4 months and 5-year OS of 41%). A meta-analysis by Helm et al. in 2015 includes

1047 patients from 20 studies with a 5-year OS of 42% [16]. Our results in the nine patients with epithelioid PM in whom CRS + HIPEC has been possible with curative intent (median OS 58 months, 5-year OS 47.4%) are therefore in the high range of the reference series. Our DFS (median 17 months, 4-year 38%), although also remarkable, underestimates the real benefit since it is calculated up to the date of the first relapse; however, a complete cytoreduction was achieved in two of the recurrences (with no subsequent relapse). Therefore, the patients free of disease at the time of data analysis are not 3 out of 9, but 5 out of 9; however, this number is not reflected in the DFS concept.

The sarcomatoid subtype has such a poor prognosis that it is actually considered a contraindication for CRS + HIPEC [7]. The prognosis of biphasic PM is worse than the epithelioid subtype; however, it is possible to increase the survival rate with complete CRS + HIPEC in properly selected patients [27]. Our study clearly demonstrates the worst prognosis of biphasic tumors, with unresectable disease and survival of less than 6 months in the three cases.

Palliative HIPEC can be used in DMPM for the treatment of malignant ascites [8,9]. In our study, six palliative HIPECs were performed (three of them laparoscopic) in three patients, with prolonged survival in two of them (both epithelioid). PIPAC, combined with systemic CT, has been used in peritoneal carcinomatosis of various origins mainly with palliative intention, leading to clinical response rates of 67–75% in DMPM [28]. However, it has never been compared with laparoscopic palliative HIPEC, which is ostensibly cheaper and surprisingly forgotten in favor of PIPAC.

Multicystic PM has a much better prognosis, is more common in women (83%), and usually has an incidental diagnosis, as reflected in our series. Traditional treatment is surgical resection, although long-term follow-up is necessary due to the high probability of recurrence (50%) and the exceptional possibility of malignant transformation [11]. CRS + HIPEC in experienced centers is considered the treatment of choice nowadays [7], and the three patients in our series (treated with CRS + HIPEC without postoperative mortality or serious complications) all remain alive and free of disease after a very long follow-up (59 months).

5. Conclusions

Our data confirm that treatment of PM with CRS + HIPEC, in correctly selected patients, seems to be the optimal treatment. It is important to know this therapeutic option, both to offer it to patients, and to avoid delays in referral to appropriate centers for treatment. CRS + HIPEC is considered a better alternative than isolated CRS also in borderline varieties of diffuse PM (well differentiated papillary and multicystic). Candidate selection should include laparoscopic staging whenever possible in DMPM. Perioperative systemic chemotherapy is indicated in certain cases, and therapeutic decisions should be made in a Multidisciplinary Tumor Board in expert centers in the treatment of peritoneal surface malignancies. Patients with unresectable disease may benefit from the use of palliative (preferably laparoscopic) HIPEC for the treatment of malignant ascites.

Author Contributions: F.P.: Conceptualization and design; acquisition, analysis, and interpretation of data; original draft preparation; final approval of the version to be published. M.P.: acquisition of data; original draft preparation. I.M., Á.S. and E.P.-V.: data collection; final approval of the version to be published. All authors have read and agreed to the published version of the manuscript, and have made a significant contribution.

Funding: This research received no external funding.

Institutional Review Board Statement: The current study was conducted in accordance with the Declaration of Helsinki, and approved by the Ethics and Clinical Research Committee of the University Hospital of Fuenlabrada, Madrid, Spain (protocol code: APR 19/27, date of approval: 27 May 2019).

Informed Consent Statement: Informed consent was obtained from all subjects involved in the study.

Data Availability Statement: All data supporting reported results are provided as part of the manuscript, and no new datasets were created.

Conflicts of Interest: The authors declare no conflict of interest.

References

1. Boffetta, P. Epidemiology of peritoneal mesothelioma: A review. *Ann. Oncol.* **2007**, *18*, 985–990. [CrossRef] [PubMed]
2. Moolgavkar, S.H.; Meza, R.; Turim, J. Pleural and peritoneal mesotheliomas in SEER: Age effects and temporal trends, 1973–2005. *Cancer Causes Control* **2009**, *20*, 935–944. [CrossRef] [PubMed]
3. Deraco, M.; Bartlett, D.; Kusamura, S.; Baratti, D. Consensus statement on peritoneal mesothelioma. *J. Surg. Oncol.* **2008**, *98*, 268–272. [CrossRef]
4. Janne, P.A.; Wozniak, A.J.; Belani, C.P.; Keohan, M.-L.; Ross, H.J.; Polikoff, J.A.; Mintzer, D.M.; Taylor, L.; Ashland, J.; Ye, Z.; et al. Open-label study of pemetrexed alone or in combination with cisplatin for the treatment of patients with peritoneal mesothelioma: Outcomes of an expanded access program. *Clin. Lung Cancer* **2005**, *7*, 40–46. [CrossRef]
5. Yan, T.D.; Deraco, M.; Baratti, D.; Kusamura, S.; Elias, D.; Glehen, O.; Gilly, F.N.; Levine, E.A.; Shen, P.; Mohamed, F.; et al. Cytoreductive surgery and hyperthermic intraperitoneal chemotherapy for malignant peritoneal mesothelioma: Multi-institutional experience. *J. Clin. Oncol.* **2009**, *27*, 6237–6242. [CrossRef]
6. Greenbaum, A.; Alexander, H.R. Peritoneal mesothelioma. *Transl. Lung Cancer Res.* **2020**, *9* (Suppl. S1), S120–S132. [CrossRef] [PubMed]
7. Kusamura, S.; Kepenekian, V.; Villeneuve, L.; Lurvink, R.; Govaerts, K.; De Hingh, I.; Moran, B.; Van der Speeten, K.; Deraco, M.; Glehen, O.; et al. Peritoneal mesothelioma: PSOGI/EURACAN clinical practice guidelines for diagnosis, treatment and follow-up. *Eur. J. Surg. Oncol.* **2021**, *47*, 36–59. [CrossRef]
8. Valle, M.; Van der Speeten, K.; Garofalo, A. Laparoscopic hyperthermic intraperitoneal peroperative chemotherapy (HIPEC) in the management of refractory malignant ascites: A multi-institutional retrospective analysis in 52 patients. *J. Surg. Oncol.* **2009**, *100*, 331–334. [CrossRef]
9. Facchiano, E.; Risio, D.; Kianmanesh, R.; Msika, S. Laparoscopic hyperthermic intraperitoneal chemotherapy: Indications, aims, and results: A systematic review of the literature. *Ann. Surg. Oncol.* **2012**, *19*, 2946–2950. [CrossRef]
10. Vogin, G.; Network, T.R.; Hettal, L.; Vignaud, J.-M.; Dartigues, P.; Goere, D.; Ferron, G.; Heyd, B.; Bereder, J.-M.; Tuech, J.-J.; et al. Well-Differentiated Papillary Mesothelioma of the Peritoneum: A Retrospective Study from the RENAPE Observational Registry. *Ann. Surg. Oncol.* **2019**, *26*, 852–860. [CrossRef]
11. Noiret, B.; Renaud, F.; Piessen, G.; Eveno, C. Multicystic peritoneal mesothelioma: A systematic review of the literature. *Pleura Peritoneum* **2019**, *4*, 20190024. [CrossRef] [PubMed]
12. Sugarbaker, P.H.; Chang, D. Long-term regional chemotherapy for patients with epithelial malignant peritoneal mesothelioma results in improved survival. *Eur. J. Surg. Oncol.* **2017**, *43*, 1228–1235. [CrossRef]
13. Baratti, D.; Kusamura, S.; Cabras, A.D.; Bertulli, R.; Hutanu, I.; Deraco, M. Diffuse malignant peritoneal mesothelioma: Long-term survival with complete cytoreductive surgery followed by hyperthermic intraperitoneal chemotherapy (HIPEC). *Eur. J. Cancer* **2013**, *49*, 3140–3148. [CrossRef] [PubMed]
14. Gomez Portilla, A.; Cendoya, I.; Muriel, J.; Olabarria, I.; Guede, N.; Moraza, N.; Fernández, E.; Martínez de Lecea, C.; Magrach, L.; Martín, E.; et al. Malignant peritoneal mesothelioma. Our experienced with triple combined therapy: Cytoreduction, intraperitoneal perioperative chemotherapy and hyperthermia. *Cir. Esp.* **2007**, *81*, 82–86. [CrossRef] [PubMed]
15. Alexander, H.R., Jr.; Bartlett, D.L.; Pingpank, J.F.; Libutti, S.K.; Royal, R.; Hughes, M.S.; Holtzman, M.; Hanna, N.; Turner, K.; Beresneva, T.; et al. Treatment factors associated with long-term survival after cytoreductive surgery and regional chemotherapy for patients with malignant peritoneal mesothelioma. *Surgery* **2013**, *153*, 779–786. [CrossRef]
16. Helm, J.H.; Miura, J.T.; Glenn, J.A.; Marcus, R.K.; Larrieux, G.; Jayakrishnan, T.T.; Donahue, A.E.; Gamblin, T.C.; Turaga, K.K.; Johnston, F.M. Cytoreductive surgery and hyperthermic intraperitoneal chemotherapy for malignant peritoneal mesothelioma: A systematic review and meta-analysis. *Ann. Surg. Oncol.* **2015**, *22*, 1686–1693. [CrossRef]
17. Dindo, D.; Demartines, N.; Clavien, P.A. Classification of surgical complications: A new proposal with evaluation in a cohort of 6336 patients and results of a survey. *Ann. Surg.* **2004**, *240*, 205–213. [CrossRef]
18. Seshadri, R.A.; Hemanth Raj, E. Diagnostic Laparoscopy in the Pre-operative Assessment of Patients Undergoing Cytoreductive Surgery and HIPEC for Peritoneal Surface Malignancies. *Indian J. Surg. Oncol.* **2016**, *7*, 230–235. [CrossRef]
19. Passot, G.; Dumont, F.; Goéré, D.; Arvieux, C.; Rousset, P.; Regimbeau, J.; Elias, D.; Villeneuve, L.; Glehen, O.; Abba, J.; et al. Multicentre study of laparoscopic or open assessment of the peritoneal cancer index (BIG-RENAPE). *Br. J. Surg.* **2018**, *105*, 663–667. [CrossRef]
20. Chua, T.C.; Yan, T.D.; Saxena, A.; Morris, D.L. Should the treatment of peritoneal carcinomatosis by cytoreductive surgery and hyperthermic intraperitoneal chemotherapy still be regarded as a highly morbid procedure?: A systematic review of morbidity and mortality. *Ann. Surg.* **2009**, *249*, 900–907.
21. Malgras, B.; Gayat, E.; Aoun, O.; Lo Dico, R.; Eveno, C.; Pautrat, K.; Delhorme, J.B.; Passot, G.; Marchal, F.; Sgarbura, O.; et al. Impact of Combination Chemotherapy in Peritoneal Mesothelioma Hyperthermic Intraperitoneal Chemotherapy (HIPEC): The RENAPE Study. *Ann. Surg. Oncol.* **2018**, *25*, 3271–3279. [CrossRef] [PubMed]

22. Deraco, M.; Baratti, D.; Hutanu, I.; Bertuli, R.; Kusamura, S. The role of perioperative systemic chemotherapy in diffuse malignant peritoneal mesothelioma patients treated with cytoreductive surgery and hyperthermic intraperitoneal chemotherapy. *Ann. Surg. Oncol.* **2013**, *20*, 1093–1100. [CrossRef] [PubMed]
23. Kepenekian, V.; Elias, D.; Passot, G.; Mery, E.; Goere, D.; Delroeux, D.; Quenet, F.; Ferron, G.; Pezet, D.; Guilloit, J.M.; et al. Diffuse malignant peritoneal mesothelioma: Evaluation of systemic chemotherapy with comprehensive treatment through the RENAPE Database: Multi-Institutional Retrospective Study. *Eur. J. Cancer* **2016**, *65*, 69–79. [CrossRef] [PubMed]
24. Le Roy, F.; Gelli, M.; Hollebecque, A.; Honoré, C.; Boige, V.; Dartigues, P.; Benhaim, L.; Malka, D.; Ducreux, M.; Elias, D.; et al. Conversion to Complete Cytoreductive Surgery and Hyperthermic Intraperitoneal Chemotherapy for Malignant Peritoneal Mesothelioma After Bidirectional Chemotherapy. *Ann. Surg. Oncol.* **2017**, *24*, 3640–3646. [CrossRef] [PubMed]
25. Alyami, M.; Mercier, F.; Siebert, M.; Bonnot, P.E.; Laplace, N.; Villeneuve, L.; Passot, G.; Glehen, O.; Bakrin, N.; Kepenekian, V. Unresectable peritoneal metastasis treated by pressurized intraperitoneal aerosol chemotherapy (PIPAC) leading to cytoreductive surgery and hyperthermic intraperitoneal chemotherapy. *Eur. J. Surg. Oncol.* **2021**, *47*, 128–133. [CrossRef]
26. Sgarbura, O.; Gourgou, S.; Tosi, D.; Bakrin, N.; Bouazza, N.; Delaine, S.; De Forges, H.; Pocard, M.; Quénet, F. MESOTIP: Phase II multicenter randomized trial evaluating the association of PIPAC and systemic chemotherapy vs. systemic chemotherapy alone as 1st-line treatment of malignant peritoneal mesothelioma. *Pleura Peritoneum* **2019**, *4*, 20190010. [CrossRef]
27. Votanopoulos, K.I.; Sugarbaker, P.; Deraco, M.; Morris, D.; Glehen, O.; Elias, D.; De Simone, M.; Robella, M.; Heyd, B.; Kusamura, S.; et al. Is Cytoreductive Surgery with Hyperthermic Intraperitoneal Chemotherapy Justified for Biphasic Variants of Peritoneal Mesothelioma? Outcomes from the Peritoneal Surface Oncology Group International Registry. *Ann. Surg. Oncol.* **2018**, *25*, 667–673. [CrossRef]
28. Alyami, M.; Hübner, M.; Grass, F.; Bakrin, N.; Villeneuve, L.; Laplace, N.; Passot, G.; Glehen, O.; Kepenekian, V. Pressurised intraperitoneal aerosol chemotherapy: Rationale, evidence, and potential indications. *Lancet Oncol.* **2019**, *20*, e368–e377. [CrossRef]

Journal of
Clinical Medicine

MDPI

Article

Treatment of Peritoneal Surface Malignancies by Cytoreductive Surgery (CRS) and Hyperthermic Intraperitoneal Chemotherapy (HIPEC) in Spain: Results of the National Registry of the Spanish Group of Peritoneal Oncologic Surgery (REGECOP)

Israel Manzanedo [1,2,3,*], Fernando Pereira [1,2,3], Pedro Cascales-Campos [3,4], Cristobal Muñoz-Casares [3,5], Enrique Asensio [3,6], Juan Torres-Melero [3,7], Arancha Prada-Villaverde [3,8], Ibán Caravaca-García [3,9], Alberto Gutiérrez-Calvo [3,10], Javier Vaqué [3,11], Gloria Ortega [3,12], Alberto Titos-García [3,13], Laura González-Sánchez [3,14], Estíbalitz Pérez-Viejo [1,2,3], Ángel Serrano [1,2,3], Beatriz Martínez-Torres [1,2,3] and REGECOP Group †

1 Peritoneal Carcinomatosis Unit, Department of General and Digestive Surgery, Hospital Universitario de Fuenlabrada, 28942 Madrid, Spain; fernando.pereira@salud.madrid.org (F.P.); estibalitz.perez@salud.madrid.org (E.P.-V.); aserranom@salud.madrid.org (Á.S.); bmartinezt@salud.madrid.org (B.M.-T.)
2 Department of Surgery, Rey Juan Carlos University (URJC), 28933 Madrid, Spain
3 Spanish Group of Peritoneal Oncologic Surgery (GECOP), 28001 Madrid, Spain; cascalescirugia@gmail.com (P.C.-C.); fcocris@gmail.com (C.M.-C.); easensiodi@saludcastillayleon.es (E.A.); juantorresmelero@gmail.com (J.T.-M.); aranchaprada@hotmail.com (A.P.-V.); ivan_med06@hotmail.com (I.C.-G.); alberto.gutierrez@salud.madrid.org (A.G.-C.); fjvaque@yahoo.es (J.V.); gortega@mdanderson.es (G.O.); albertotitosg@hotmail.com (A.T.-G.); lgsanchez08@gmail.com (L.G.-S.)
4 Peritoneal Oncologic Surgery Unit, Department of Surgery, Hospital Virgen de la Arrixaca, IMIB-ARRIXACA, 30120 Murcia, Spain
5 Department of Surgery, Hospital Virgen del Rocío, 41013 Sevilla, Spain
6 Advanced Oncologic Surgery Unit, Department of General and Digestive Surgery, Hospital Río Hortega, 47012 Valladolid, Spain
7 Department of General and Digestive Surgery, Hospital Universitario de Torrecárdenas, 04009 Almería, Spain
8 Department of General and Digestive Surgery, Hospital Infanta Cristina, 06080 Badajoz, Spain
9 Department of General and Digestive Surgery, Hospital General Universitario de Elche, 03203 Alicante, Spain
10 Department of General and Digestive Surgery, Hospital Príncipe de Asturias de Alcalá de Henares, 28805 Madrid, Spain
11 Department of General and Digestive Surgery, Hospital de La Fe, 46026 Valencia, Spain
12 Department of General and Digestive Surgery, Hospital MD Anderson Cancer Center, 28033 Madrid, Spain
13 Department of General and Digestive Surgery, Hospital Regional Universitario de Málaga, 29010 Málaga, Spain
14 Department of General and Digestive Surgery, Hospital Insular, 35016 Las Palmas de Gran Canaria, Spain
* Correspondence: israel.manzanedo@salud.madrid.org; Tel.: +34-91-6006266
† Collaborators of Register of Spanish Group of Peritoneal Oncologic Surgery (REGECOP) indicated in Acknowledgements section.

Abstract: Introduction: Treatment of Peritoneal Surface Malignancies (PSM) with cytoreductive surgery (CRS) and hyperthermic intraperitoneal chemotherapy (HIPEC) has achieved results never seen before in these patients, which classically have a poor prognosis. The possibility of conducting clinical trials in these diseases is complicated, since some of them are rare, so the analysis of large databases provides very valuable scientific information. The aim of this study is to analyze the global results of the National Registry of the Spanish Group of Peritoneal Oncologic Surgery (REGECOP), whose objective is to register all patients scheduled for HIPEC nationwide. Methods: This is a retrospective analysis of the data recorded in the REGECOP from 36 Spanish hospitals from 2001 to 2021. There were 4159 surgical interventions in 3980 patients. Results: 66% are women and 34% are men with a median age of 59 years (range 17–86). 41.5% of the patients were treated for Peritoneal Metastases (PM) of colorectal cancer (CRC); 32.4% were women with ovarian cancer (OC) with PM; 12.8% were treated for pseudomyxoma peritonei (PMP); 6.2% had PM from gastric cancer (GC); 4.9% had PM of non-conventional origin; and, finally, 2.1% of cases were patients diagnosed with peritoneal mesothelioma. The median Peritoneal Cancer Index (PCI) was 9 (0–39), and complete cytoreduction was achieved in 81.7% of the procedures. Severe morbidity (Dindo–Clavien grade III–IV) was observed in 17.7% of surgeries, with 2.1% mortality. Median hospital stay was 11 days (0–259). Median overall survival (OS) was 41 months for CRC patients, 55 months for women with OC, was not reached in PMP patients, was 14 months for GC patients, and 66 months in mesothelioma patients. Conclusions: large databases provide extremely useful data. CRS with HIPEC in referral centers is a safe treatment with encouraging oncologic results in PSM.

Keywords: peritoneal carcinomatosis; HIPEC; cytoreductive surgery; Peritoneal Surface Malignancies

1. Introduction

Peritoneal Surface Malignancies (PSM) are a heterogeneous group of primary tumors like primary peritoneal carcinoma or peritoneal mesothelioma, and peritoneal metastases (PM) from other abdominopelvic tumors by cell dissemination, such as from colon, stomach, or ovarian cancer, or pseudomyxoma peritonei secondary to appendiceal mucinous neoplasia [1,2].

Classically, PSM were considered as terminal diseases and therefore were paired with supportive care and palliative treatments. Since the end of the twentieth century, and especially since the beginning of the twenty-first century, progress has been made in the knowledge of the peritoneum and its diseases, and today PSM are considered as local dissemination that can be treated, in selected cases, with radical intent [3].

The combination of modern systemic chemotherapy with cytoreductive surgery (CRS) and hyperthermic intraperitoneal chemotherapy (HIPEC) is achieving very encouraging results and is already considered the standard treatment in some indications, such as peritoneal pseudomyxoma (PMP) or peritoneal mesothelioma [4,5]; in other indications, such as PM from colorectal, ovarian, or gastric cancers, there is more discussion regarding CRS with HIPEC, but the published studies show promising results [6–10].

The scientific evidence on this treatment is growing. However, there are few multicenter randomized clinical trials, because carrying them out is very difficult, since some of these diseases are very rare and make the recruitment of patients very difficult. For this reason, national prospective registries of large patient series are of great importance in clarifying the potential benefit of these procedures and their real risks.

The Spanish Group of Peritoneal Oncologic Surgery (GECOP) was born in 2007 and gathers all the centers where CRS and HIPEC procedures are performed in Spain. It is currently made up by 39 centers. One of the objectives of the GECOP since its foundation was the creation of a prospective registry of patients treated through CRS and HIPEC. However, it was not until 2020 that this goal became a total reality and the National Registry of the Spanish Group of Peritoneal Oncologic Surgery (REGECOP) began to be fully operational. The objective of this article is to analyze the overall results of the REGECOP.

2. Patients and Methods

This is a retrospective, multicenter study from a prospective national database of patients with PSM of different origins scheduled for treatment with CRS and HIPEC from 2001 to 2021. Both patients with PSM and patients at high risk of developing PM and who had undergone second-look surgery with prophylactic HIPEC were included. An intention-to-treat analysis was carried out. The study was approved by the ethics committee in each participating center.

All participating centers are members of the GECOP and are specialized in the treatment of peritoneal oncological disease. Depending on the number of procedures performed, the centers were divided into 2 groups: high-volume centers if they have performed more than 100 procedures or low-volume centers if they have performed less than 100. The high-volume centers are described in Table 1. A total of 36 centers participated in the study.

Table 1. Centers with more than 100 procedures (high-volume centers).

Hospital	Region	Number of Procedures
H. Universitario de Fuenlabrada	Madrid	735
H. Virgen de la Arrixaca	Murcia	369
H. Virgen del Rocío	Sevilla	271
H. Río Hortega	Valladolid	210
H. Torrecárdenas	Almería	202
H. Infanta Cristina	Badajoz	147
H. General de Elche	Alicante	136
H. Príncipe de Asturias	Madrid	135
H. La Fe	Valencia	129
MD Anderson	Madrid	119
H. Regional de Málaga	Málaga	115
H. Insular	Gran Canaria	102

The extension of peritoneal disease is established according to the Peritoneal Cancer Index (PCI) [11], and the radicality of CRS is assessed by the Completeness of Cytoreduction Score (CCS) [12]. CRS is considered a high-complexity surgery when more than 4 visceral resections or peritonectomies have been performed. Data about HIPEC itself is also collected, such as type of perfusion technique (open close, or close with CO_2 recirculation), drug used, or administration time.

Postoperative morbidity is classified according to Dindo–Clavien classification [13], and complications grade III or IV are considered as severe morbidity. Hospital stay is defined as the days between date of surgery and date of discharge.

During surveillance, recurrences and deaths are registered. Reverse Kaplan–Meier was used to calculate median follow-up. Disease-free survival (DFS) is defined as the time between the date of surgery and the date of first relapse or death. Overall survival (OS) is defined as the time from the date of surgery to death.

The statistical analysis was performed using IBM SPSS software, version 22.0. Outcome analysis was performed using the Chi square test, *t* test, Mann–Whitney *U* test, and contingency tables. Kaplan–Meier curves were used for survival analysis, the log rank test to identify difference between curves, and Cox multiple regression analysis to investigate possible prognostic factors; $p \leq 0.05$ is considered significant.

3. Results

The 36 centers have registered 4159 procedures in 3980 patients. Repeated CRS with HIPEC was performed in 155 patients: 136 were operated on twice, 15 received CRS and HIPEC three times, 3 patients were operated on four times, and 1 patient five times. Major preoperative, surgical, and postoperative characteristics of the 4159 procedures are summarized in Table 2. A comparison was made between high- and low-volume centers, which is shown in Table 3.

Table 2. Preoperative, surgical, and postoperative characteristics.

Variable	Procedures (n = 4159)
Sex (%)	
Female	65.8
Male	34.2
Median age (years (range))	59 (18–86)
Primary tumor (%)	
Colorectal cancer	41.4
Ovarian cancer	31.9
Pseudomyxoma peritonei	13.3

Table 2. *Cont.*

Variable	Procedures (n = 4159)
Gastric cancer	6
Peritoneal mesothelioma	2.6
Non-conventional indications	4.8
Neoadjuvant SCT (%)	63.2
Laparoscopic surgery (%)	2.7
Median surgical PCI (range)	9 (0–39)
High-complexity surgery (%)	41.4
CCS (%)	
CCS-0	81.7
CCS-1	7.5
CCS-2	2.2
CCS-3	8.6
HIPEC technique (%)	
Open or coliseum	69.2
Close	3.5
Close with CO_2 recirculation	27.3
HIPEC drug (%)	
MMC	34.3
Oxaliplatin	24.5
Paclitaxel	18
Cisplatin	10.8
Cisplatin + Doxorubicin	8.4
Cisplatin + MMC	2.5
Others	1.6
Postoperative complications (%)	
No complication	49.9
Minor (I–II)	30.3
Severe complications (III–IV)	17.7
Grade V	2.1
Surgical reintervention (%)	11.9
Median hospital stay (days (range))	11 (0–259)

SCT, systemic chemotherapy; PCI, Peritoneal Cancer Index; CCS, Completeness of Cytoreduction Score; MMC, mitomycin C.

Table 3. Comparison of high- and low-volume centers.

Variable	High-Volume Center	Low-Volume Center	p
Median surgical PCI (range)	9 (0–39)	8 (0–39)	0.001
CCS (%)			
CCS-0 or CCS-1	89.4	88.9	0.36
CCS-2 or CCS-3	10.6	11.1	
Postoperative complications (%)			
No complication	52.8	44.8	
Minor (I–II)	27.5	35.3	0.0001
Severe complications (III–IV)	17.7	17.5	
Grade V	2	2.4	
Median disease-free survival (months)	16	15	0.49
Median overall survival (months)	47	49	0.48

PCI, Peritoneal Cancer Index; CCS, Completeness of Cytoreduction Score.

3.1. Colorectal Cancer

Colorectal Cancer is the most frequent indication in this registry, with 1716 procedures in 1647 patients. Median age of the patients is 60 years (18–86), with 46.1% women and 53.9% men. Peritoneal relapses (metachronous PM) of a previously operated colorectal cancer constitute 50.8% of the procedures. Preoperative systemic chemotherapy (SCT) was administered in 58.1% of patients. The median surgical PCI is 6 (0–39); 65% of patients have a PCI lower than 10 and 10.8% have a PCI of 20 or higher. Complete cytoreduction (CCS-0) was achieved in 85.5% of surgeries, with a rate of high-complexity surgeries of 32.9%. The most-used drug in HIPEC was mitomycin C (MMC) in 55.2% of cases, followed by oxaliplatin with 41.4%; since June 2018, the use of oxaliplatin dropped significantly, going from being the majority with 56.1% of HIPEC to being used only in 17.2% of cases since then ($p < 0.05$). Severe morbidity occurred in 18.8% of cases, surgical reintervention was necessary in 14.5%, and mortality was 2.5%. The use of oxaliplatin was associated with significant increased severe morbidity (26.2%) compared to the use of MMC (14.4%), accompanied by a higher risk of mortality (4% versus 1.3%, $p < 0.05$). Median hospital stay is 12 days (1–195). With a median follow-up of 37 months, median DFS is 13 months (3-year DFS of 23.9% and 5-year DFS of 17.5%) and median OS is 41 months (3-year OS of 55.7% and 5-year OS of 35.6%) (Figure 1). According to the PCI, median OS is 53 months for a PCI of 0-10, 34 months for a PCI of 11–15, 21 months for a PCI of 16–20, and 10 months for a PCI higher than 20 ($p = 0.0001$) (Figure 2).

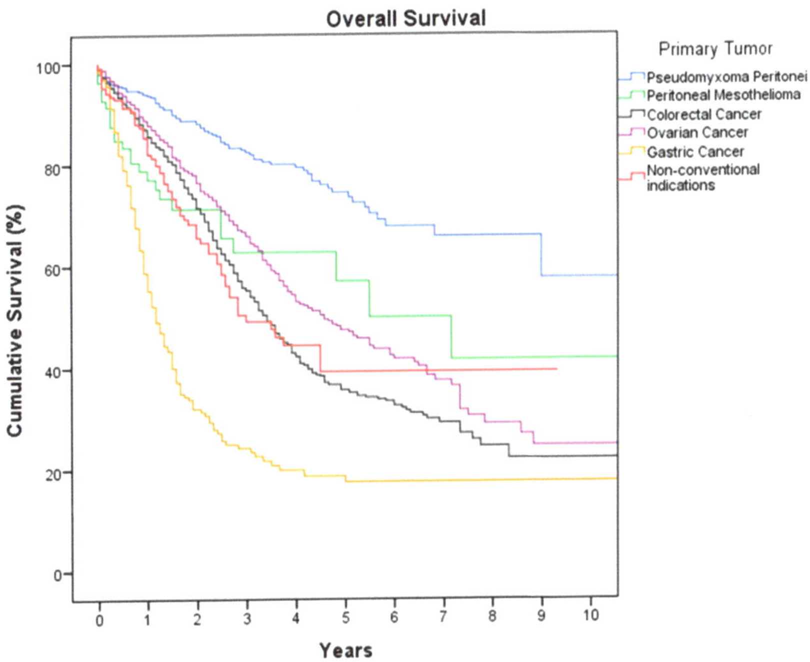

Figure 1. Overall survival of patients treated with cytoreductive surgery and HIPEC according to tumoral origin.

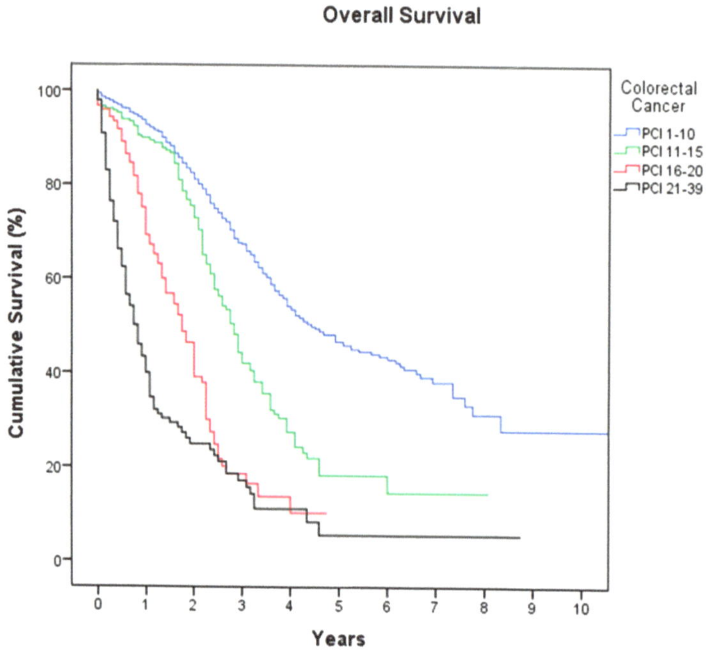

Figure 2. Overall Survival in colorectal cancer according to Peritoneal Cancer Index (PCI).

3.2. Ovarian Cancer

One thousand three hundred twenty-four CRS and HIPEC procedures were performed in 1285 patients with ovarian cancer and PM. The median age is 59 years (20–85). The majority of procedures are primary cytoreductions (68.1%), with 31.9% being secondary cytoreductions (relapses surgery). Upfront surgery (CRS without neoadjuvant SCT) was carried out in 10% of primary cytoreductions; 90% of primary cytoreductions were interval surgeries (CRS after neoadjuvant SCT). The median PCI is 11 (0–39); 23.7% of cases have a PCI higher than 20. Complete cytoreduction (CCS-0) was achieved in 82.4% of cases and CCS-1 in 9.4%, with a rate of high-complexity surgeries of 54.6%. The most-used HIPEC drug was paclitaxel (52.9%), followed by cisplatin (38.9%). Severe complications were observed in 15.6% of patients, and 9.1% of patients were reoperated on in the postoperative period; postoperative mortality was 1.3%. The median hospital stay is 10 days (1–160). The median follow-up is 34 months. The median DFS is 16 months (3-year DFS of 31.1% and 5-year DFS of 24.1%). The median OS is 55 months (3-year OS of 66.7% and 5-year OS of 47.4%) (Figure 1). Median OS in patients with a PCI of 0-20 was 66 months, and it was 29 months in those with a PCI higher than 20 ($p = 0.0001$). Complete cytoreduction (CCS-0 and CCS-1) is a good prognostic factor of OS, with a median OS of 62 months versus 12 months with incomplete CRS (CCS-2 or CCS-3) ($p = 0.0001$).

3.3. Pseudomyxoma Peritonei (PMP)

Five hundred and fifty CRS and HIPEC procedures were carried out in 508 patients diagnosed with PMP. Median age of the patients is 60 years (18–85), with 58.9% women. The median PCI is 14 (0–39), significantly higher than the other indications (median PCI of 8, $p < 0.05$); furthermore, 39% of patients have extensive disease, with a PCI greater than 20. Complete cytoreduction (CCS-0) was achieved in 76.1% of surgeries, and nearly complete cytoreduction (CCS-1) in 13.1%. High-complexity surgery was necessary in 47.2% of CRSs. MMC is the HIPEC drug most commonly used (62.6%), followed by oxaliplatin (30.4%). Severe morbidity was observed in 19.7% of cases, with a 13.3% reoperation rate in the postoperative period; postoperative mortality is 3.6%. The median hospital stay is 12 days (0–259). The median surveillance is 33 months. The median DFS is 68 months (5-year DFS of 51.9%), and the median OS was not reached (5-year OS of 74.4%) (Figure 1).

3.4. Gastric Cancer

Two hundred and fifty procedures of CRS and HIPEC were performed in 246 patients with gastric cancer. The median age of the patients is 56 years (21–84), with 46.2% women and 53.8% men. Neoadjuvant SCT was administered in 89% of patients. The median PCI is 6 (0–39), and 76% of patients have a PCI lower than 12. Complete cytoreduction (CCS-0) was achieved in 77.3% of surgeries, with a high-complexity surgery rate of 41.2%. The HIPEC drug most commonly used was cisplatin alone or in combination with other drugs (61.6%). Severe morbidity was observed in 19% of cases, with 1.7% mortality; the surgical reintervention rate is 10.1%. The median hospital stay is 12 days (1–228). The median follow-up is 40 months. The median DFS is 7 months (3-year DFS of 15.1% and 5-year DFS of 12.3%). The median OS is 14 months (3-year OS of 24.2% and 5-year OS of 18.7%) (Figure 1); the median OS reaches 20 months for a PCI of 0-6 with a 5-year OS of 28%, while for a PCI higher than 6, the median OS falls to 9 months with a 5-year OS of 2.6% ($p = 0.0001$) (Figure 3).

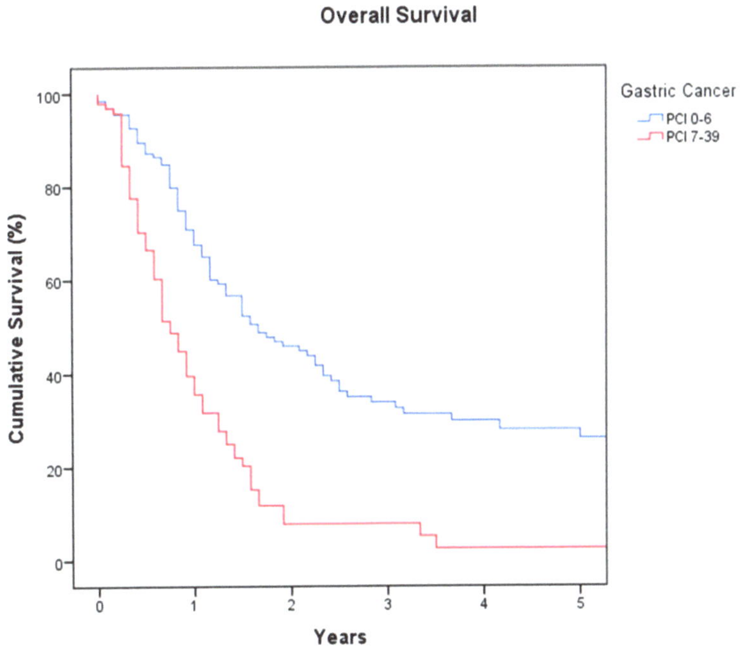

Figure 3. Overall survival in gastric cancer according to Peritoneal Cancer Index (PCI).

3.5. Peritoneal Mesothelioma

One hundred and seven procedures were performed in 90 patients diagnosed with peritoneal mesothelioma. Patients' median age is 54 years (18–83), with 59.8% women. The median PCI is significantly higher than other indications (20 versus 8, $p < 0.05$), with a PCI $\geq$ 20 in 51.4% of cases. Complete or nearly complete cytoreduction (CCS-0 or CCS-1) was achieved in 74.2% of CRSs. High-complexity surgery was necessary in 59.6% of CRSs. Cisplatin (alone or in combination) is the HIPEC drug most used (85.3%). Severe complications occurred in 16.8% of cases, with an 11.1% surgical reintervention rate; postoperative mortality is 2.8%. The median hospital stay is 11.5 days (1–142). The median follow-up is 23 months. The median DFS is 11 months (3-year DFS of 27.2%), and the median OS is 66 months (3-year OS of 62.7%) (Figure 1).

3.6. Non-Conventional Indications

One hundred and ninety-nine CRS and HIPEC procedures were carried out in 194 patients. The origins were very diverse, with the most frequent being endometrial and small bowel cancer, non-mucinous appendix neoplasms, or sarcomas. The median age is 56 years (18–81), with 68.8% women. The median PCI is 9 (0–39). Complete cytoreduction (CCS-0) was reached in 81.6% of CRSs, with a high-complexity surgery rate of 42.3%. Severe morbidity was registered in 14.9% of cases, and the mortality rate was 0.5%. Median hospital stay is 10 days (1–67). The OS results are shown in Figure 1: the median DFS is 12 months (5-year DFS of 20.9%), and the median OS is 36 months (5-year OS of 39.2%).

4. Discussion

The management of PSM has changed in recent years, from being terminal diseases with a poor prognosis to diseases with curative treatment possibilities in selected cases. CRS associated with HIPEC have achieved encouraging results in different tumoral origins. However, the medical community remains skeptical and critical of this treatment due to the few published randomized clinical trials to date, although several clinical trials have been published and multiple studies are ongoing [6–9,14–18]. Currently CRS with HIPEC is considered the standard treatment only for PMP and peritoneal mesothelioma, curiously two pathologies where there are no published clinical trials because they are rare diseases [19,20]. While scientific evidence continues to grow, national prospective registries with large numbers of patients can contribute to clarify the benefit of these procedures and their efficacy by analyzing morbidity and mortality.

This study shows the results of a large database of Spanish centers. It is one of the studies with the largest number of patients that have been published to date. The main indications are colorectal cancer and ovarian cancer (more than 70%), because these are the most prevalent diseases. Despite the fact that surgical technique is demanding, with a high-complexity surgery rate greater than 40% to achieve a high percentage of complete cytoreductions (81.7%), serious morbidity is quite acceptable, with 17.7%, and 2.1% mortality. Although morbidity is lower in high-volume centers (Table 3), this improvement is at the expense of mild complications, as severe morbidity in low-volume centers is also acceptable. These results are remarkable compared to published studies. In a recent study, Ramos et al. described 20% of severe complications in 1321 consecutive CRS + HIPEC procedures [21]. In 2022, Filis et al. published a meta-analysis in ovarian cancer; they observed 143 adverse events in 308 patients (46.4%) treated with CRS and HIPEC [22]. The PRODIGE 7 trial, published in 2021, registered severe morbidity in 42% of patients in the CRS plus HIPEC group [6].

Colorectal cancer is the most common origin of PM. In the beginning of the 21st century, Verwaal et al. published the first clinical trial of PM of colorectal cancer origin [23]; they randomized 105 patients to receive standard treatment with SCT or aggressive cytoreduction and HIPEC. The median OS in the HIPEC group was significantly higher than the standard group (22.3 months versus 12.6, $p = 0.032$). These results meant a big change, and CRS with HIPEC began to be considered as a treatment option in selected patients. In 2008, the same authors published an update of the trial with more years of follow-up, which confirmed the results obtained in the first study [15]. However, many medical oncologists considered the Verwaal trial quickly outdated since the SCT used in it became obsolete coinciding with the time of the first publication, son, in any case, it would be necessary to make a comparison with the newer drugs (oxaliplatin, irinotecan, cetuximab, and bevacizumab). To answer these questions, the PRODIGE 7 study was carried out; Quenet et al. randomized 265 patients in two groups (CRS alone versus CRS + HIPEC), and the median OS was similar in both groups (41.7 months in the CRS group and 41.2 in the CRS + HIPEC group) [6]. The results of PRODIGE 7 shows that selected patients with PM of colorectal cancer origin must be operated on, because CRS achieves a median OS longer than 3 years, better than what is achieved with SCT, but the addition of oxaliplatin HIPEC is not shown to increase survival; the role of HIPEC is in question, and future studies are necessary to know its value. HIPEC can prevent peritoneal recurrence in locally advanced colorectal cancer, according to a recent trial [24], but its efficacy for the treatment of peritoneal metastases will be evaluated in ongoing studies [7]. The results of the REGECOP demonstrate the efficacy of CRS and HIPEC, with a median OS of 41 months and a 5-year OS of 35.6%; even if patients have a PCI of 10 or lower, the median OS reaches 53 months. Since the results of the PRODIGE 7 study were shown in 2018 in an ASCO meeting, there has been a change in the trend in the REGECOP groups, with using MMC more frequently with the use of oxaliplatin being almost anecdotal at present. On the other hand, our study shows greater severe complications with the use of oxaliplatin. For these reasons, the GECOP group is currently conducting a clinical trial using HIPEC with MMC [7], and currently the HIPEC scheme with oxaliplatin should only be used within clinical trials in view of the results.

Patients with ovarian cancer frequently develop PM, and the use of HIPEC has been controversial. This study shows a median OS of 55 months with a 5-year OS of 47.4%. The most important prognostic factors are the PCI and the quality of cytoreduction according to the CCS; the median OS for a PCI of 0–20 is 66 months (29 months in PCI 21–39), and the median OS is 62 months for CCS-0 or CCS-1 versus 12 months in CCS-2 or CCS-3. The CRS is a standard of care in ovarian cancer, but the use of HIPEC is discussed. Spiliotis et al., in 2015, published a clinical trial for recurrent ovarian cancer; the addition of HIPEC improved OS (3-year OS of 75% versus 18%) in 120 randomized patients [14], but this trial was widely criticized for its methodology. In 2018, Van Driel et al. randomized 245 patients with stage III ovarian cancer, after induction of SCT, to receive interval CRS with or without HIPEC; HIPEC improved median OS (48 versus 34 months) with comparable severe morbidity in both groups [8]. These results are comparable to the trial of Cascales-Campos et al. published in 2022, with an improvement in median OS from 45 months in the non-HIPEC group to 52 months in the HIPEC group without morbidity differences [18]. Despite all the scientific evidence, the gynecologic oncology community remains reluctant to use HIPEC. According to the evidence of these trials and a recent meta-analysis published [22], in primary ovarian cancer the interval CRS with HIPEC is a safe option that improves DFS and OS.

Pseudomyxoma peritonei (PMP) is a rare peritoneal disease originated from a mucinous neoplasm of the appendix. PMP incidence is estimated at around one to three cases per million each year. CRS with HIPEC is the standard treatment with good results. Our study shows the best survival results in PMP despite the fact that the volume of peritoneal disease was high (median PCI of 14), with a DFS of 68 months (5-year DFS of 51.9%) and the median OS not reached (5-year OS of 74.4%). These results are similar to different published studies. In 2021, Kusamura et al. published the results of 1924 patients from the Peritoneal Surface Oncologic Group International (PSOGI) registry; patients treated with CRS and HIPEC had a 5-year OS of 57.8%, better than the patients treated with CRS alone (5-year OS 46.2%) [25]. In 2021, an international consensus was published where bases on the diagnosis and treatment of PMP were founded, establishing CRS and HIPEC as its standard treatment [19].

Gastric cancer with PM has a poor prognosis, with a median OS of 6 months and a 5-year OS of 0% [26]. However, treatment with CRS and HIPEC in selected cases obtains encouraging results. In 2011, a randomized clinical trial was published with 68 patients randomized to CRS and HIPEC or CRS alone; patients treated with HIPEC had significantly better survival (median OS of 11 months versus 6.5 months) [9]. This is the only clinical trial published to date, but there are numerous high-quality studies heading in the same direction. Bonnot et al. published the CYTO-CHIP study in 2019, a propensity score study that compared 180 patients treated with CRS and HIPEC with 97 patients treated with surgery alone; median OS was higher in the HIPEC group (18.8 months versus 12.1), without differences in morbidity or mortality [10]. Furthermore, several meta-analyses showed similar results, with a robust benefit of treatment with CRS and HIPEC [27–30]. The results of the REGECOP show a median OS of 14 months (5-year OS of 18.7%); if the PCI is lower than 7, the median OS is 20 months (5-year OS 28%). Patient selection is essential to obtain the best results, and experts currently recommend a PCI limit of 12 or even 7 to perform an aggressive treatment with CRS and HIPEC [26,31,32].

Peritoneal mesothelioma is the other established indication for CRS and HIPEC in addition to PMP [20]. In 2013, Baratti et al. published a series of 108 patients with peritoneal mesothelioma treated with CRS and HIPEC with a median OS of 63.2 months [33]. Helm et al. published an important meta-analysis including 1407 patients, and they observed a 5-year OS of 42% [34]. The median OS for peritoneal mesothelioma in our study is 66 months, similar to published studies.

CRS and HIPEC have been used in other non-conventional indications. These have included a miscellany of diverse origins, such as endometrial cancer, small bowel cancer, or sarcomas. This heterogeneity of pathologies makes it impossible to make an analysis of survival, but it is possible to draw conclusions about the safety of the procedure according to morbidity. In the present study, severe morbidity was observed in 4.9% of cases, and the mortality rate was 0.5%. Retrospective studies have been published evaluating the use of CRS and HIPEC as treatment for PM of non-conventional origins. In 2022, Rajha et al. showed the results of 76 patients with PM arising from infrequent tumor entities, with a median OS of 68 months [35]. CRS with HIPEC can be a treatment option for selected patients with PM of different origins.

Despite the obvious limitations of a non-randomized, non-experimental, and solely observational study, this is a study with a large number of patients that provides great information. While waiting for the results of important clinical trials in progress, large national series, such as the present REGECOP study, can be very useful. With the results obtained in this study, we can affirm that CRS with HIPEC is a safe treatment for patients with PSM, which achieves very good outcomes if it is performed in experienced centers. In the coming years, the scientific evidence will increase as different ongoing trials are published [7,17]. Meanwhile, it is very important that these patients are evaluated and treated in expert centers and following the recommendations of different guidelines and consensus [19,20,36–38].

5. Conclusions

The REGECOP study confirms that treatment with CRS + HIPEC is a safe option for selected patients with PSM. The survival results are remarkable and similar to previously published studies. It is one of the series with the largest number of patients published to date, so our results add highly valid and real information about patients treated in Spain. CRS with HIPEC is the treatment that provides the greatest survival today for patients with PSM. All patients diagnosed with PSM should be referred to experienced centers.

Author Contributions: I.M.: Conceptualization and design; acquisition, analysis, and interpretation of data; original draft preparation; final approval of the version to be published. F.P.: acquisition of data; original draft preparation; final approval of the version to be published. E.P.-V., Á.S. and B.M.-T.: final approval of the version to be published. P.C.-C., C.M.-C., E.A., J.T.-M., A.P.-V., I.C.-G., A.G.-C., J.V., G.O., A.T.-G. and L.G.-S.: acquisition of data. REGECOP group: conceptualization; project administration; acquisition of data. All authors have read and agreed to the published version of the manuscript.

Funding: This research was financed by Combat Medical LTD.

Institutional Review Board Statement: The current study was conducted in accordance with the Declaration of Helsinki and approved by the Ethics and Clinical Research Committee of Hospital Universitario Príncipe de Asturias, Alcalá de Henares, Madrid, Spain (protocol code: REG-COP-2020-01, date of approval: 1 July 2020).

Informed Consent Statement: Informed consent was obtained from all subjects involved in the study.

Data Availability Statement: The data used to support the findings of the present study are available from the corresponding author upon request.

Acknowledgments: This study has been possible thanks to the collaboration of all centers that participate in the REGECOP. The other collaborators of the REGECOP group not included among the authors are as follows: Javier Lacueva from Hospital General de Elche, Alicante; Remedios Gómez Sanz from Hospital Príncipe de Asturias de Alcalá de Henares, Madrid; Domenico Sabia from Hospital Sant Joan Despi Mosses Broggi, Barcelona; Eduardo Díaz Reques from Hospital Sanchinarro, Madrid; Manuel Artiles Armas from Hospital Doctor Negrín, Las Palmas de Gran Canaria; Susana Sánchez García from Hospital Universitario de Ciudad Real; Marta Roldón Golet from Hospital Quirón, Málaga; Pere Bretxa from Hospital Quirón Torrevieja, Alicante; Estrella Turienzo from Hospital Central de Asturias, Oviedo; Araceli Mayol Oltra from Consorcio Hospitalario Provincial de Castellón; María Isabel Prieto from Hospital Universitario de La Paz, Madrid; Xabier Arteaga from Hospital Universitario Donosti, San Sebastián; Julio Galindo Álvarez from Hospital Ramón y Cajal, Madrid; Alfonso García Fadrique from Instituto Valenciano de Oncología, Valencia; Natividad Palencia García from Hospital Gregorio Marañón, Madrid; Emilio Terol Garaulet from Hospital General Reina Sofía, Murcia; Álvaro Arjona Sánchez from Hospital Reina Sofía, Córdoba; Rosa María Álvarez Seoane from Complejo Hospitalario Universitario de A Coruña; Vanessa Concepción Martín from Hospital Nuestra Señora de la Candelaria, Santa Cruz de Tenerife; Vicente Borrego Estella from Hospital Clínico Lozano Blesa, Zaragoza; Pedro Villarejo Campos from Fundación Jiménez Díaz, Madrid; Cristina Pineño from Hospital Son Espases, Palma de Mallorca; Manuel Marcello Fernández from Fundación Alcorcón, Madrid; Cristina Rihuete Caro from Hospital Infanta Elena, Valdemoro, Madrid; Fernando López Mozos from Hospital Clínico de Valencia; and Fernando Martínez Regueira from Clínica Universitaria de Navarra, Pamplona.

Conflicts of Interest: The authors declare no conflict of interest. The REGECOP is supported by COMBAT. Role of the funding source: support in data collection; the funders had no role in the design of the study, in the interpretation of data, in the writing of the manuscript, or in the decision to publish the results.

References

1. Brücher, B.L.; Piso, P.; Verwaal, V.; Esquivel, J.; Derraco, M.; Yonemura, Y.; Gonzalez-Moreno, S.; Pelz, J.; Königsrainer, A.; Ströhlein, M.; et al. Peritoneal carcinomatosis: Cytoreductive surgery and HIPEC—Overview and basics. *Cancer Investig.* **2012**, *30*, 209–224. [CrossRef] [PubMed]
2. Bhatt, A.; Glehen, O. Extent of Peritoneal Resection for Peritoneal Metastases: Looking Beyond a Complete Cytoreduction. *Ann. Surg. Oncol.* **2020**, *27*, 1458–1470. [CrossRef]
3. Yonemura, Y.; Canbay, E.; Li, Y.; Coccolini, F.; Glehen, O.; Sugarbaker, P.H.; Morris, D.; Moran, B.; Gonzaletz-Moreno, S.; Deraco, M.; et al. A comprehensive treatment for peritoneal metastases from gastric cancer with curative intent. *Eur. J. Surg. Oncol.* **2016**, *42*, 1123–1131. [CrossRef] [PubMed]
4. Yan, T.D.; Welch, L.; Black, D.; Sugarbaker, P.H. A systematic review on the efficacy of cytoreductive surgery combined with perioperative intraperitoneal chemotherapy for diffuse malignancy peritoneal mesothelioma. *Ann. Oncol.* **2007**, *18*, 827–834. [CrossRef] [PubMed]
5. Sugarbaker, P.H. New standard of care for appendiceal epithelial neoplasms and pseudomyxoma peritonei syndrome? *Lancet Oncol.* **2006**, *7*, 69–76. [CrossRef] [PubMed]
6. Quénet, F.; Elias, D.; Roca, L.; Goéré, D.; Ghouti, L.; Pocard, M.; Facy, O.; Arvieux, C.; Lorimier, G.; Pezet, D.; et al. Cytoreductive surgery plus hyperthermic intraperitoneal chemotherapy versus cytoreductive surgery alone for colorectal peritoneal metastases (PRODIGE 7): A multicentre, randomised, open-label, phase 3 trial. *Lancet Oncol.* **2021**, *22*, 256–266. [CrossRef]
7. Pereira, F.; Serrano, A.; Manzanedo, I.; Pérez-Viejo, E.; González-Moreno, S.; González-Bayón, L.; Arjona-Sánchez, A.; Torres, J.; Ramos, I.; Barrios, M.E.; et al. GECOP-MMC: Phase IV randomized clinical trial to evaluate the efficacy of hyperthermic intraperitoneal chemotherapy (HIPEC) with mytomicin-C after complete surgical cytoreduction in patients with colon cancer peritoneal metastases. *BMC Cancer* **2022**, *22*, 536. [CrossRef]
8. van Driel, W.J.; Koole, S.N.; Sikorska, K.; Schagen van Leeuwen, J.H.; Schreuder, H.W.R.; Hermans, R.H.M.; de Hingh, I.H.J.T.; van der Velden, J.; Arts, H.J.; Massuger, L.F.A.G.; et al. Hyperthermic Intraperitoneal Chemotherapy in Ovarian Cancer. *N. Engl. J. Med.* **2018**, *378*, 230–240. [CrossRef]
9. Yang, X.-J.; Huang, C.-Q.; Suo, T.; Mei, L.-J.; Yang, G.-L.; Cheng, F.-L.; Zhou, Y.-F.; Xiong, B.; Yonemura, Y.; Li, Y. Cytoreductive surgery and hyperthermic intraperitoneal chemotherapy improves survival of patients with peritoneal carcinomatosis from gastric cancer: Final results of a phase III randomized clinical trial. *Ann. Surg. Oncol.* **2011**, *18*, 1575–1581. [CrossRef]
10. Bonnot, P.-E.; Piessen, G.; Kepenekian, V.; Decullier, E.; Pocard, M.; Meunier, B.; Bereder, J.-M.; Abboud, K.; Marchal, F.; Quenet, F.; et al. Cytoreductive Surgery With or Without Hyperthermic Intraperitoneal Chemotherapy for Gastric Cancer With Peritoneal Metastases (CYTO-CHIP study): A Propensity Score Analysis. *J. Clin. Oncol.* **2019**, *37*, 2028–2040. [CrossRef]

11. Portilla, A.G.; Shigeki, K.; Dario, B.; Marcello, D. The intraoperative staging systems in the management of peritoneal surface malignancy. *J. Surg. Oncol.* **2008**, *98*, 228–231. [CrossRef]
12. González-Moreno, S.; Kusamura, S.; Baratti, D.; Deraco, M. Postoperative residual disease evaluation in the locoregional treatment of peritoneal surface malignancy. *J. Surg. Oncol.* **2008**, *98*, 237–241. [CrossRef]
13. Dindo, D.; Demartines, N.; Clavien, P.-A. Classification of surgical complications: A new proposal with evaluation in a cohort of 6336 patients and results of a survey. *Ann. Surg.* **2004**, *240*, 205–213. [CrossRef] [PubMed]
14. Spiliotis, J.; Halkia, E.; Lianos, E.; Kalantzi, N.; Grivas, A.; Efstathiou, E.; Giassas, S. Cytoreductive surgery and HIPEC in recurrent epithelial ovarian cancer: A prospective randomized phase III study. *Ann. Surg. Oncol.* **2015**, *22*, 1570–1575. [CrossRef]
15. Verwaal, V.J.; Bruin, S.; Boot, H.; van Slooten, G.; van Tinteren, H. 8-year follow-up of randomized trial: Cytoreduction and hyperthermic intraperitoneal chemotherapy versus systemic chemotherapy in patients with peritoneal carcinomatosis of colorectal cancer. *Ann. Surg. Oncol.* **2008**, *15*, 2426–2432. [CrossRef] [PubMed]
16. Glehen, O.; Passot, G.; Villeneuve, L.; Vaudoyer, D.; Bin-Dorel, S.; Boschetti, G.; Piaton, E.; Garofalo, A. GASTRICHIP: D2 resection and hyperthermic intraperitoneal chemotherapy in locally advanced gastric carcinoma: A randomized and multicenter phase III study. *BMC Cancer* **2014**, *14*, 183. [CrossRef]
17. Noiret, B.; Piessen, G.; Eveno, C. Update of randomized controlled trials evaluating cytoreductive surgery (CRS) and hyperthermic intraperitoneal chemotherapy (HIPEC) in prevention and therapy of peritoneal metastasis: A systematic review. *Pleura Peritoneum* **2022**, *7*, 51–61. [CrossRef] [PubMed]
18. Antonio, C.C.P.; Alida, G.G.; Elena, G.G.; Rocío, G.S.; Jerónimo, M.G.; Luis, A.R.J.; Aníbal, N.D.; Francisco, B.V.; Jesús, G.R.Á.; Pablo, R.R.; et al. Cytoreductive Surgery With or Without HIPEC After Neoadjuvant Chemotherapy in Ovarian Cancer: A Phase 3 Clinical Trial. *Ann. Surg. Oncol.* **2022**, *29*, 2617–2625. [CrossRef]
19. Govaerts, K.; Lurvink, R.J.; De Hingh, I.; Van der Speeten, K.; Villeneuve, L.; Kusamura, S.; Kepenekian, V.; Deraco, M.; Glehen, O.; Moran, J.; et al. Appendiceal tumours and pseudomyxoma peritonei: Literature review with PSOGI/EURACAN clinical practice guidelines for diagnosis and treatment. *Eur. J. Surg. Oncol.* **2021**, *47*, 11–35. [CrossRef]
20. Kusamura, S.; Kepenekian, V.; Villeneuve, L.; Lurvink, R.J.; Govaerts, K.; De Hingh, I.; Moran, B.J.; Van der Speeten, K.; Deraco, M.; Glehen, O.; et al. Peritoneal mesothelioma: PSOGI/EURACAN clinical practice guidelines for diagnosis, treatment and follow-up. *Eur. J. Surg. Oncol.* **2021**, *47*, 36–59. [CrossRef]
21. Bernadó, M.I.R.; Maña, O.C.; Martín-Baranera, M.; Sánchez, P.B. Morbimortality after 1321 consecutive CRS + HIPEC procedures: Seeking excellence in surgery for peritoneal surface malignancy. *Clin. Transl. Oncol.* 2023; *Online ahead of print*. [CrossRef]
22. Filis, P.; Mauri, D.; Markozannes, G.; Tolia, M.; Filis, N.; Tsilidis, K. Hyperthermic intraperitoneal chemotherapy (HIPEC) for the management of primary advanced and recurrent ovarian cancer: A systematic review and meta-analysis of randomized trials. *ESMO Open* **2022**, *7*, 100586. [CrossRef] [PubMed]
23. Verwaal, V.J.; van Ruth, S.; de Bree, E.; van Sloothen, G.W.; van Tinteren, H.; Boot, H.; Zoetmulder, F.A.N. Randomized trial of cytoreduction and hyperthermic intraperitoneal chemotherapy versus systemic chemotherapy and palliative surgery in patients with peritoneal carcinomatosis of colorectal cancer. *J. Clin. Oncol.* **2003**, *21*, 3737–3743. [CrossRef]
24. Arjona-Sánchez, A.; Espinosa-Redondo, E.; Gutiérrez-Calvo, A.; Segura-Sampedro, J.J.; Pérez-Viejo, E.; Concepción-Martín, V.; Sánchez-García, S.; García-Fadrique, A.; Prieto-Nieto, I.; Barrios-Sanchez, P.; et al. Efficacy and Safety of Intraoperative Hyperthermic Intraperitoneal Chemotherapy for Locally Advanced Colon Cancer: A Phase 3 Randomized Clinical Trial. *JAMA Surg.* **2023**, e230662. [CrossRef]
25. Kusamura, S.; Barretta, F.; Yonemura, Y.; Sugarbaker, P.H.; Moran, B.J.; Levine, E.A.; Goere, D.; Baratti, D.; Nizri, E.; Morris, D.L.; et al. The Role of Hyperthermic Intraperitoneal Chemotherapy in Pseudomyxoma Peritonei After Cytoreductive Surgery. *JAMA Surg.* **2021**, *156*, e206363. [CrossRef] [PubMed]
26. Manzanedo, I.; Pereira, F.; Pérez-Viejo, E.; Serrano, Á. Gastric Cancer with Peritoneal Metastases: Current Status and Prospects for Treatment. *Cancers* **2023**, *15*, 1777. [CrossRef]
27. Desiderio, J.; Chao, J.; Melstrom, L.; Warner, S.; Tozzi, F.; Fong, Y.; Parisi, A.; Woo, Y. The 30-year experience—A meta-analysis of randomised and high-quality non-randomised studies of hyperthermic intraperitoneal chemotherapy in the treatment of gastric cancer. *Eur. J. Cancer* **2017**, *79*, 1–14. [CrossRef]
28. Granieri, S.; Bonomi, A.; Frassini, S.; Chierici, A.P.; Bruno, F.; Paleino, S.; Kusamura, S.; Germini, A.; Facciorusso, A.; Deraco, M.; et al. Prognostic impact of cytoreductive surgery (CRS) with hyperthermic intraperitoneal chemotherapy (HIPEC) in gastric cancer patients: A meta-analysis of randomized controlled trials. *Eur. J. Surg. Oncol.* **2021**, *47*, 2757–2767. [CrossRef]
29. Zhang, J.-F.; Lv, L.; Zhao, S.; Zhou, Q.; Jiang, C.-G. Hyperthermic Intraperitoneal Chemotherapy (HIPEC) Combined with Surgery: A 12-Year Meta-Analysis of this Promising Treatment Strategy for Advanced Gastric Cancer at Different Stages. *Ann. Surg. Oncol.* **2022**, *29*, 3170–3186. [CrossRef]
30. Martins, M.; Santos-Sousa, H.; Araújo, F.; Nogueiro, J.; Sousa-Pinto, B. Impact of Cytoreductive Surgery with Hyperthermic Intraperitoneal Chemotherapy in the Treatment of Gastric Cancer with Peritoneal Carcinomatosis: A Systematic Review and Meta-analysis. *Ann. Surg. Oncol.* **2022**, *29*, 7528–7537. [CrossRef]
31. Glehen, O.; Gilly, F.N.; Arvieux, C.; Cotte, E.; Boutitie, F.; Mansvelt, B.; Bereder, J.M.; Lorimier, G.; Quenet, F.; Elias, D.; et al. Peritoneal carcinomatosis from gastric cancer: A multi-institutional study of 159 patients treated by cytoreductive surgery combined with perioperative intraperitoneal chemotherapy. *Ann. Surg. Oncol.* **2010**, *17*, 2370–2377. [CrossRef]

32. Chia, C.S.; You, B.; Decullier, E.; Vaudoyer, D.; Lorimier, G.; Abboud, K.; Bereder, J.-M.; Arvieux, C.; Boschetti, G.; Glehen, O.; et al. Patients with Peritoneal Carcinomatosis from Gastric Cancer Treated with Cytoreductive Surgery and Hyperthermic Intraperitoneal Chemotherapy: Is Cure a Possibility? *Ann. Surg. Oncol.* **2016**, *23*, 1971–1979. [CrossRef]
33. Baratti, D.; Kusamura, S.; Cabras, A.D.; Bertulli, R.; Hutanu, I.; Deraco, M. Diffuse malignant peritoneal mesothelioma: Long-term survival with complete cytoreductive surgery followed by hyperthermic intraperitoneal chemotherapy (HIPEC). *Eur. J. Cancer* **2013**, *49*, 3140–3148. [CrossRef]
34. Helm, J.H.; Miura, J.T.; Glenn, J.A.; Marcus, R.K.; Larrieux, G.; Jayakrishnan, T.T.; Donahue, A.E.; Gamblin, T.C.; Turaga, K.K.; Johnston, F.M. Cytoreductive surgery and hyperthermic intraperitoneal chemotherapy for malignant peritoneal mesothelioma: A systematic review and meta-analysis. *Ann. Surg. Oncol.* **2015**, *22*, 1686–1693. [CrossRef]
35. Rajha, A.; Piso, P.; Halmy, L.; Panczel, I.; Nedelcut, D.-S.; Herold, Z.; Szasz, A.M.; Acs, M. Rare Histologies and Infrequent Indications for Cytoreductive Surgery and Hyperthermic Intraperitoneal Chemotherapy. *Anticancer. Res.* **2022**, *42*, 3681–3692. [CrossRef]
36. Kusamura, S.; Bhatt, A.; Hubner, M.; Villeneuve, L.; Deraco, M.; Bakrin, N.; Van Der Speeten, K.; Glehen, O. The 2022 PSOGI International Consensus on HIPEC Regimens for Peritoneal Malignancies: Methodology. *Ann. Surg. Oncol.* **2023**, *30*, 2508–2519. [CrossRef] [PubMed]
37. van Stein, R.M.; Lok, C.A.; Aalbers, A.G.; de Hingh, I.H.; Houwink, A.P.; Stoevelaar, H.J.; Sonke, G.S.; van Driel, W.J. Standardizing HIPEC and perioperative care for patients with ovarian cancer in the Netherlands using a Delphi-based consensus. *Gynecol. Oncol. Rep.* **2022**, *39*, 100945. [CrossRef] [PubMed]
38. Chicago Consensus Working Group; Izquierdo, F.J.; Schuitevoerder, D.; Plana, A.; Eng, O.S.; Sherman, S.; Badgwell, B.; Johnston, F.M.; Abdel-Misih, S.; Blazer, D.G.; et al. The Chicago Consensus on Peritoneal Surface Malignancies: Management of Gastric Metastases. *Cancer* **2020**, *126*, 2541–2546. [CrossRef]

Journal of
Clinical Medicine

MDPI

Article

Simultaneous Surgical Approach with Hyperthermic Intraperitoneal Chemotherapy (HIPEC) in Patients with Concurrent Peritoneal and Liver Metastases of Colon Cancer Origin

Rafael Morales-Soriano [1,2,3,4,*], Cristina Pineño-Flores [1,2], José Miguel Morón-Canis [1], Francisco Javier Molina-Romero [1,2], José Carlos Rodriguez-Pino [1], Julia Loyola-Miró [1], Francisco Xavier Gonzalez-Argente [1,2,3], Elías Palma-Zamora [1], Mónica Guillot-Morales [5], Sandra Giménez [5], Melchor Alvarez-Mon [6], Miguel A. Ortega [6] and Juan José Segura-Sampedro [1,2,3]

1 Department of Digestive Surgery, University Hospital Son Espases, 07120 Palma de Mallorca, Spain; cristina.pineno@ssib.es (C.P.-F.); josem.moron@ssib.es (J.M.M.-C.); xmolina@ssib.es (F.J.M.-R.); josec.pino@ssib.es (J.C.R.-P.); julia.loyola@ssib.es (J.L.-M.); xavier.gonzalez@ssib.es (F.X.G.-A.); eliasf.palma@ssib.es (E.P.-Z.); juan.segura@ssib.es (J.J.S.-S.)

2 Faculty of Medicine, University of the Balearic Islands, 07122 Palma de Mallorca, Spain

3 Health Research Institute of the Balearic Islands (IDISBA), 07120 Palma de Mallorca, Spain

4 Royal Academy of Medicine of the Balearic Islands, 07120 Palma de Mallorca, Spain

5 Department of Medical Oncology, University Hospital Son Espases, 07120 Palma de Mallorca, Spain; monicam.guillot@ssib.es (M.G.-M.); sandra.gimenez@ssib.es (S.G.)

6 Department of Medicine and Medical Specialties, Faculty of Medicine and Health Sciences (IRYCIS), University of Alcalá, 28801 Alcalá de Henares, Spain; mademons@gmail.com (M.A.-M.); miguel.angelortega92@gmail.com (M.A.O.)

* Correspondence: rafa.morales@telefonica.net

Abstract: Background: Simultaneous liver resection and peritoneal cytoreduction with hyperthermic intraperitoneal chemotherapy (HIPEC) remains controversial today. The aim of the study was to analyze the postoperative outcomes and survival of patients with advanced metastatic colon cancer (peritoneal and/or liver metastases). **Methods:** Retrospective observational study from a prospective maintained data base. Patients who underwent a simultaneous peritoneal cytoreduction and liver resection plus HIPEC were studied. Postoperative outcomes and overall and disease free survival were analyzed. Univariate and multivariate analyses were performed. **Results:** From January 2010 to October 2022, 22 patients operated with peritoneal and liver metastasis (LR+) were compared with 87 patients operated with peritoneal metastasis alone (LR−). LR+ group presented higher serious morbidity (36.4 vs. 14.9%; p: 0.034). Postoperative mortality did not reach statistical difference. Median overall and disease free survival was similar. Peritoneal carcinomatosis index was the only predictive factor of survival. **Conclusions**: Simultaneous peritoneal and liver resection is associated with increased postoperative morbidity and hospital stay, but with similar postoperative mortality and OS and disease free survival. These results reflect the evolution of these patients, considered inoperable until recently, and justify the trend to incorporate this surgical strategy within a multimodal therapeutic plan in highly selected patients.

Keywords: HIPEC; colon cancer; liver metastases; peritoneal carcinomatosis; combined resection

1. Introduction

In the last two decades, the appearance of new cytostatics and biological agents, together with the improvement of perioperative care and surgical technique, has changed the prognosis of metastatic colon cancer. Surgical resection of liver metastases, applied in more than 30% of patients, has achieved 5-year survival rates around 40% [1,2] and something similar has occurred with the surgical resection of isolated pulmonary metastases [2,3].

Peritoneal metastases are the metastatic form with the worst prognosis, being the second cause of death in colon cancer, probably due to the lower penetration of cytostatics in the peritoneal nodules [4]. However, some studies have reported fairly similar survival results between patients with liver metastases and those with peritoneal metastases [5,6].

It is estimated that approximately 8% of patients with colon cancer develop hepatic and peritoneal metastases simultaneously [1,7]. Simultaneous resection of the primary tumor together with liver metastases is now routinely performed [8], but until 1999, the concomitant presence of liver and peritoneal metastases was considered a contraindication for surgical treatment and these patients were considered unresectable and amenable only to palliative adjuvant chemotherapy, with an overall survival of 12 months [4,7]. Elias et al. and a consensus statement showed that the presence of three liver metastases with a low peritoneal tumor burden (PCI < 12) did not suppose an absolute contraindication for simultaneous treatment with CRC + HIPEC [9–11]. Since then, several studies and meta-analyses have published acceptable morbidity and mortality results, with a median survival of around 25–48 months in selected patients treated with simultaneous surgical treatment of both lesions and the administration of HIPEC and adjuvant chemotherapy [1,10–21]. Despite these publications, simultaneous resection of liver and peritoneal metastases remains controversial due to its increased morbidity, mortality, and delayed administration of adjuvant chemotherapy, and for these reasons it has not been established as the standard of care [1,2,9–11,13,15,18,19].

The aim of this study was to evaluate the impact of simultaneous liver resection and peritoneal cytoreductive surgery with HIPEC on perioperative and survival outcomes. The hypothesis was that this surgical concomitant approach would be associated with higher morbidity and/or mortality than patients with CCR-HIPEC alone.

2. Material and Methodology

2.1. Study Design and Patient Selection

This is a retrospective analysis of all consecutive patients with concurrent peritoneal and liver metastasis due to colon cancer, treated with peritoneal cytoreduction with HIPEC, in a tertiary referral hospital from January 2008 to October 2021. Two groups of patients were formed. The control group (LR−) consisted of patients who underwent cytoreduction and HIPEC alone, while the experimental group (LR+) consisted of patients who underwent peritoneal cytoreduction with simultaneous resection of liver metastases plus HIPEC. This study was approved by the Multidisciplinary Committee of Peritoneal Surface Oncologic Malignancies and the Investigation Commission of the Universitari Son Espases Hospital.

Inclusion criteria were an Eastern Cooperative Oncology Group (ECOG) score of 0–2, an American Society of Anesthesiologists (ASA) score of 0–3, peritoneal and liver resectable disease, the absence of extra-abdominal metastasis, patients younger than 75 years of age, adequate renal, bone marrow and liver function, and specific written informed consent.

Exclusion criteria were extra-abdominal or unresectable disease, poor performance status (ECOG 3–5 or ASA > 3), progressive disease after neoadjuvant chemotherapy, presence of another neoplasia, and patients having CRS and HIPEC for a Second-Look protocol. Patients with appendiceal or rectal origin were excluded from the analysis. Other exclusion criteria were a PCI higher than 17 points, patients not amenable to complete cytoreduction and lost follow-up.

Data collected. Patient demographics, medical history, and clinical data were collected and analyzed (PCI, number of organs resected, length of operation, grade of cytoreduction, stoma formation, and type of cytostatic and duration of HIPEC). Additionally, perioperative outcomes were included in the analysis (90 days morbidity according to Clavien–Dindo classification, mortality, and transfusion rate), as well as length of intensive care and hospital stay and need for reoperation. In the study, patients who experienced a relapse after undergoing the first CRS-HIPEC procedure and underwent a second CRS-HIPEC procedure were re-enrolled. The calculation of overall survival and disease-free survival (DFS) was performed differently for each procedure. For the first procedure, overall survival was calculated from the date of diagnosis to one day prior to the date of the second surgery and the patient was censored. DFS was calculated from the date of the first surgery to the date of the first recurrence. For the second procedure, overall survival was calculated from the date of the second surgery to the date of death, and DFS was calculated from the date of the second surgery to the date of the second recurrence.

Preoperative Planning. All patients were evaluated by a multidisciplinary committee on peritoneal surface malignancies and liver tumors, made up of surgeons, oncologists, radiologists and nuclear medicine physicians. Radiological evaluation was made with thoracic an abdomen-pelvis CT scan with intravenous contrast and with a positron emission tomography (PET) when indicated by the committee. Patients with liver metastasis were evaluated with hepatic nuclear magnetic resonance. When a high PCI was suspected, laparoscopy was performed to assess the possibility of complete peritoneal cytoreduction in order to avoid unnecessary laparotomies [22]. Neoadjuvant chemotherapy was administered according to the oncologist decision. Preoperative prophylactic intravenous antibiotics (cefotaxime 2 g and metronidazole 500 mg) were infused 30 min before incision and maintained over a 48-h period. Anesthetic strategy was based on general anesthesia, epidural analgesia, invasive monitoring, and goal-directed fluid balance [23].

2.2. Follow-Up

A joint follow-up was carried out by oncology and surgery units, with controls one month and three months after the intervention and subsequently every 6 months with clinical examination, CT scan and tumor markers. Postoperative chemotherapy was administered according to the oncologic team.

2.3. Operative Technique

A xifopubic incision was routinely made with the patient in the Lloyd Davies position. In patients with liver resection a transversal right flank incision was made as necessary. In all patients with liver metastasis, an intraoperative liver ultrasound was performed. Intraoperatively, volume of peritoneal disease was quantified by the peritoneal carcinomatosis index (PCI) [24] and potential complete cytoreduction was assessed. Liver resections were performed first, followed by peritoneal cytoreduction. Only infiltrated peritoneum by tumor was excised. The decision for resection was established if complete peritoneal cytoreduction and hepatic resection could be achieved. All surgical procedures were performed by experienced surgeons and were standardized to minimize variability. Cytoreductive surgery (CRS) was performed in accordance with techniques described by Bao and Bartlett to achieve CC-0 (no residual macroscopic disease) or CC-1 (residual tumor nodule < 2.5 mm) resection [25]. HIPEC was only performed in cases of optimal peritoneal resection (CC-0 and CC-1) and complete liver resection. A standard institutional protocol for HIPEC was initiated after complete CRS, with the open technique (Coliseum) and target intraperitoneal tissue temperature of 42 °C. We used oxaliplatin in colorectal cancer until 2018, then changed to mitomycin C (20 mg/m^2 for 60 min and 10 mg/m^2 for 30 min diluted in 3 L/m^2 of a 1.5% glucose solution at 42 °C). All safety measures on cytostatic management and control of possible spillages based on the recommendations of this type of procedures were applied [26,27]. Postoperative morbidity was classified according to the Clavien–Dindo grading system [28]. For the purpose of analysis, grades 3–4 were considered major complications. Postoperative morbidity and mortality were registered within 90 days of surgery.

2.4. Endpoints

Primary endpoints were postoperative mortality and severe morbidity (Clavien–Dindo grades 3–4) at 90 days. Secondary endpoints were disease free survival (DFS) and overall survival (OS). DFS was defined as the time from CRS-HIPEC to relapse or death. OS was defined as the time from CRS-HIPEC to the time of death due to any cause.

2.5. Statistical Analysis

Data are presented as the mean and standard deviation (with a 95% confidence interval), median and interquartile range, or as a percentage (%). To analyze the risks on clinical results, simple and multivariate regression techniques have been applied with the aim of eliminating possible confounding factors and estimating the adjusted effects. For immediate dichotomous results, logistic regressions have been applied and, for numerical ones, linear regressions. Clinical results dependent on follow-up time have been analyzed using COX regression. For immediate dichotomous results, logistic regressions have been applied and, for numerical ones, linear regressions. A value of $p < 0.05$ has been considered as an indicator of a significant difference. The statistical analysis has been developed by the Methodological and Statistical Support Platform of the Balearic Islands Health Research Institute. The statistical software used to analyze the data was IBM-SPSS v.26.

2.6. Financial Support

This research was coordinated by ProA Capital, Halekulani S.L., MJR. It was co-financed by the European Development Regional Fund, 'A way to achieve Europe', as well as P2022/BMD-7321 (Community of Madrid, Spain).

3. Results

3.1. Demographics and Perioperative Characteristics

Between January 2010 and October 2022, 142 consecutive patients diagnosed with peritoneal carcinomatosis due to colon cancer underwent cytoreductive surgery and HIPEC. Of these, 33 patients were excluded for different reasons (Figure 1).

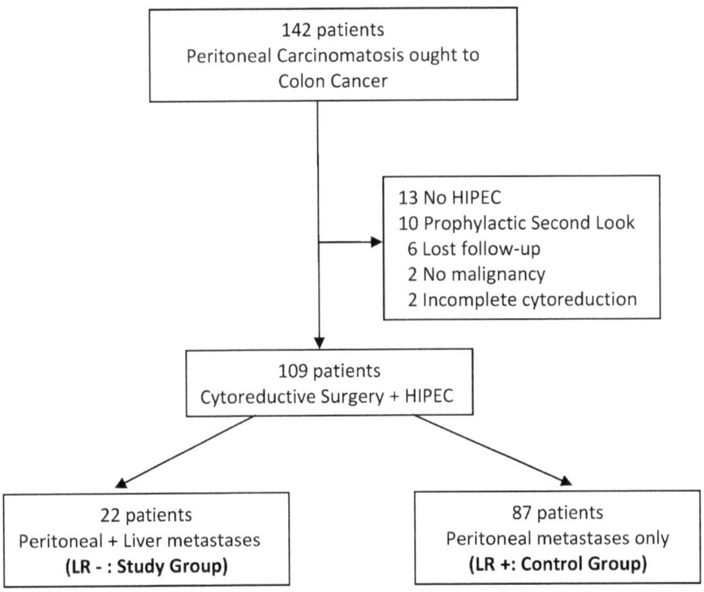

Figure 1. Study flow diagram showing patients entering in the study.

Twenty-two patients were included in the liver resection group (LR+: experimental group) and 87 patients were assigned to non-liver resection group (LR−: control group). The demographics of the study population are presented in Table 1. The LR+ group received preoperative systemic chemotherapy more frequently (40.2% vs. 54%), but without significant differences ($p = 0.226$). Variables related to surgical complexity such as PCI, operating time, organs removed, number of anastomoses, and the need for transfusion did not present significant differences. In both groups, the degree of surgical cytoreduction achieved was similar. Table 2 presents the intraoperative and histological characteristics of the liver metastases that were surgically treated. Among patients with liver metastases, the median number and size was 2 cm and 1.7, respectively, and most of them were intraparenchymal. Regarding the surgical technique, splenectomy, lateral resection of duodenum, adrenalectomy and nephrectomy were performed more frequently in LR+ (Table 3).

Table 1. Demographics and Perioperative characteristics.

Perioperative Data	LR (−) N: 87	LR (+) N: 22	p
Age	61.4 (54.9)	66.6 (60.5–71.3)	**0.030**
Female	42 (48.3%)	10 (45.5%)	0.812
Men	45 (51.7%	12 (54.5%)	
ASA-I ASA-II ASA-III	8 (9.2%) 55 (63.2%) 24 (26.4%)	3 (13.6%) 12 (54.5%) 7 (31.8%)	NA
ECOG 0 1 2 3	 52 (59.8%) 32 (36.8%) 2 (2.3%) 1 (1.1%)	 18 (81.8%) 4 (18.2%) 0 0	NA
Charlson	6 (6–7)	7 (6–8)	**0.035**
Preoperative Chemotherapy	35 (40.2%)	12 (54%)	0.226
KRAS mutation	35 (40.2%)	13 (59.1%)	0.111
Surgical PCI	8 (3–14)	9 (6–14)	0.380
Operative Time (minutes)	467 (390–567)	512 (456–638)	0.117
No. resected organs	4 (2–4)	4 (3–5)	0.171
No. of anastomosis	1 (1–3)	1 (1–3)	0.735
CCR-0 CCR-1	83 (95.4%) 4 (4.6%)	21 (95.4%) 1 (4.6%)	0.581
Transfusion rate Blood packs/patient	37 (42.5%) 1.4 (0–10)	11 (50%) 2.7 (0–12)	0.528
Stoma formation	4 (4.6%)	0	0.581

Table 2. Liver metastases characteristics.

Liver Metastases	n: 22
Location Subcapsular Intraparenchymal Both	 5 (22.7%) 15 (68.2%) 2 (9.1%)
Number of metastases 1 2 3	 9 (40.9%) 11 (50%) 2 (9.1%)
Size (cm)	2
Type of liver resection Segmentectomy Atypical resection	 9 (40.9%) 13 (59.1%)

Table 3. Types of organ resection.

Types of Resected Organ	LR (−) No (%)	LR (+) No (%)	p
Peritoneum	79 (21.9)	17 (19.9)	0.34
Omentectomy	62 (17.4)	10 (11.6)	0.06
Diaphragm resection	8 (2.2)	4 (4.6)	0.20
Gastric resection	4 (1.1)	0	0.31
Cholecystectomy	38 (10.7)	13 (15.1)	0.15
Splenectomy	16 (4.5)	0	**0.03**
Duodenum (lateral resection)	0	3 (3.5)	**0.0004**
Pancreatectomy (corporo-caudal)	3 (0.8)	0	0.38
Adrenalectomy	0	1 (1.2)	**0.004**
Small bowel	33 (9.3)	8 (9.3)	1
Right/Transverse colectomy	30 (8.5)	7 (8.1)	0.91
Left/Sigmoid/Rectal resection	36 (10.1)	10 (11.6)	0.63
Subtotal colectomy	5 (1.4)	0	0.26
Nephrectomy	0	3 (3.5)	**0.0004**
Ureter resection	6 (1.7)	2 (2.3)	0.68
Cystectomy	2 (1.1)	1 (1.2)	0.54
Hysterectomy/Ovarian resection	23 (6.5)	4 (4.6)	0.48
Aortic Lymphadenectomy	10 (2.8)	3 (3.5)	0.82

3.2. *Morbidity and Mortality*

The overall rate of complications was higher in the LR+ group (p: 0.024). The LR+ group also had more severe complications (Clavien–Dindo grades III–IV) (54.5% vs. 19.5%; p: 0.017). The distribution by type of complications was mostly similar, however, the LR+ group presented a higher incidence of abdominal abscesses (36.4% vs. 14.9%; p: 0.034). Although the incidence of postoperative pneumonia was similar, respiratory distress was significantly higher in the LR+ group (36.4% vs. 4.6%; $p < 0.001$). The second more frequent complication was intraabdominal abscesses; it is worth noting that of these infections, five of the eight (62.5%) corresponded to abscesses in the hepatectomy bed. There were no differences in the reoperation rate (Table 4). Univariate analysis showed age, transfusion, and surgical time as predictors of severe complications. However, resection of liver metastases and perioperative transfusion were the only predictor factors in multivariate analysis (Table 5). Three deaths were recorded in the overall series (2.7%), all of them belonging to the LR− group. The causes of death were respiratory failure secondary to bilateral nosocomial pneumonia with respiratory distress in two patients and one haemophagocytic syndrome with massive hemoperitoneum, most likely associated to intraperitoneal oxaliplatin. As happened with intensive care stay, hospital stay was significantly longer in the LR+ group (16 vs. 11 days; p: 0.035). A multivariate analysis of predisposing factors for postoperative mortality could not be performed due to the small number of patients.

Table 4. Morbidity and Mortality.

Postoperative Complications	LR (−) N: 87	LR (+) N: 22	
Overall Morbidity (90 days)	22 (25.3%)	11 (50%)	**0.024**
Clavien–Dindo (90 days)			
Grade 0	14 (17.7%)	5 (13.5%)	
Grade 1	15 (19%)	2 (5.4%)	
Grade 2	33 (41.8%)	15 (40.5%)	0.059
Grade 3	6 (7.6%)	5 (13.5%)	
Grade 4	9 (11.4%)	10 (27%)	**0.017**
Reinterventions	5 (5.7%)	2 (9.1%)	0.567
-Evisceration	2	0	
-Colonic fistulae	1	0	
-Abdominal abscess	1	0	
-Anastomotic dehiscence	1	1	
-Ileus	0	1	
Overall Mortality (90 days)	3 (2.7%)		
Mortality 90 (days)	3 (3.4%)	0 (0)	1.000
Causes of death			
-Bilateral Pneumonia and distress	2	0	
-Hemophagocytic syndrome	1	0	
ICU length of stay (median)	2 (2–3)	3 (2–4)	**0.039**
Hospital length of stay (median)	11 (9–16)	16 (10–35)	**0.035**
Abdominal abscess	13 (14.9%)	8 (36.4%)	**0.034**
Superficial SSI	10 (11.5%)	4 (8.2%)	0.475
Small bowel fistula	3 (3.4%)	1 (4.5%)	1.000
Anastomotic leak	2 (2.3%)	1 (4.5%)	0.495
Hemoperitoneum	2 (2.3%)	1 (4.5%)	0.495
Chylous ascites	0	1 (4.5%)	0.202
Hemothorax	1 (1.1%)	0	1.000
Thrombocytopenia	19 (21.8%)	9 (40.9%)	0.067
Ileus	11 (12.6%)	6 (27.3%)	0.106
Leukopenia	8 (9.2%)	1 (4.5%)	0.683
Pneumoniae	8 (9.2%)	3 (13.6%)	0.691
Pleural effusion with drainage	4 (4.6%)	2 (9.1%)	0.599
Pneumonia and respiratory distress	4 (4.6%)	8 (36.4%)	**0.001**
Central line sepsis	3 (3.4%)	0	1.000
Urinary infection	3 (3.4%)	1 (4.5%)	1.000
Stroke	2 (2.3%)	1 (4.5%)	0.495
Ulcerative gastritis	2 (2.3%)	0	1.000
Acute pancreatitis	1 (1.1%)	0	1.000

Table 5. Predictive factors for Severe Complications (III–IV Clavien–Dindo).

Variables	OR Crude	p	OR Adjusted	p
Liver metastases	4.29 (1.61–11.46)	**0.004**	4.36 (1.41–13.50)	**0.011**
Transfusion	3.25 (1.36–7.74)	**0.008**	3.36 (1.23–9.21)	**0.019**
Age	1.13 (0.57–2.23)	0.658	0.99 (0.98–1.01)	0.438
ASA	1.13 (0.57–2.23)	0.722	1.14 (0.53–2.44)	0.722
ECOG	0.51 (0.22–1.20)	0.124	0.72 (0.29–1.82)	0.494
PCI	1.02 (0.96–1.09)	0.533	0.99 (0.90–1.08)	0.747
Neoadjuvant chemotherapy	1.35 (0.58–3.11)	0.484	1.14 (0.44–2.96)	0.785
Operative time	1.00 (1.00–1.01)	0.112	1.00 (1.00–1.01)	0.644

3.3. Survival and Recurrence

Throughout the study period, a total of 82 patients (75.2%) presented some type of recurrence, with no differences between the two groups. The LR+ group presented a significantly higher liver recurrence (27.8 vs. 10.9%; p: 0.049). Median overall survival and DFS of the entire group was 32.4 $\pm$ 2.226 and 10.4 $\pm$ 0.966 months, respectively. Both groups had no significant differences in overall and DFS survival. The LR+ group registered a higher overall survival (43.8 vs. 30.8 months) (Table 6). Survival at one, three and five years was also similar in the two groups. Only the PCI was shown to be a predictor of overall survival (Figures 2 and 3).

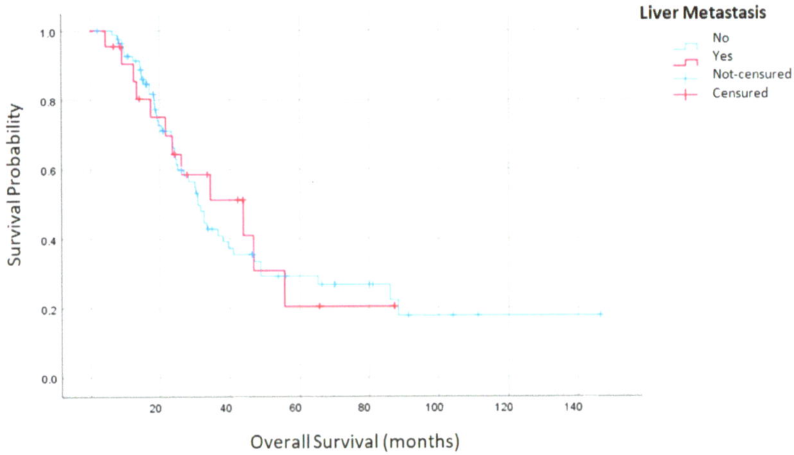

Figure 2. Overall survival of liver plus peritoneal metastases and peritoneal metastasis alone.

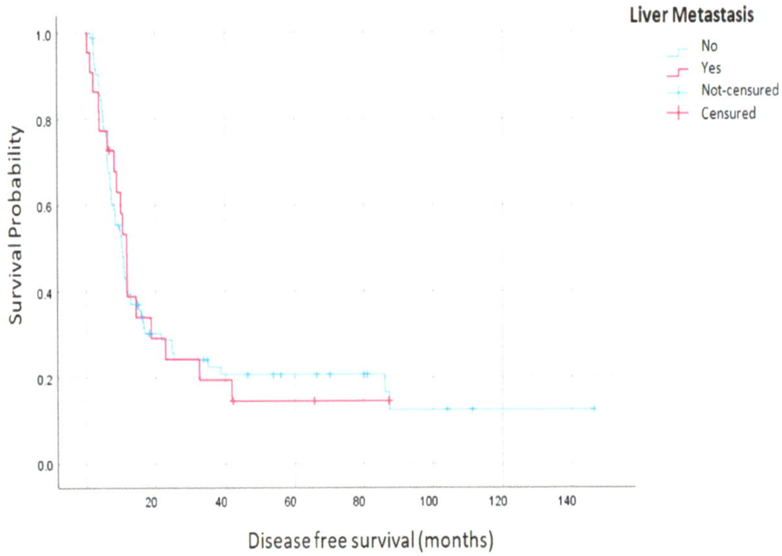

Figure 3. Disease free survival of liver plus peritoneal metastases and peritoneal metastasis alone.

Table 6. Survival.

Survival	LR (−) N: 87	LR (+) N: 22	p
Median Overall Survival	30.8 ± 2.223	43.8 ± 13.373	0.905
1 year	92%	90%	
3 years	37.7%	43.8%	
5 years	21.1%	14.3%	
Median Disease Free Survival	10.5 ± 1.257	11.7 ± 1.297	0.938
1 year	40%	38%	
3 years	22%	14%	
5 years	16%	14%	

Predictors factors of DFS were PCI and neoadjuvant chemotherapy (Table 7). The recurrence was similar in both groups (64 patients, 73.6% in LR− group and 18 patients, 81.8% in LR+ group) (p: 0.43). All recurrence sites were similar in both groups, except for liver recurrence, which was significantly higher in the LR+ group (five patients, 27.8% in LR+ group and seven patients, 10.9% in LR+ group) (p: 0.049).

Table 7. Predictive factors of survival.

Survival Predictive Factors		Univariate Analysis		Multivariate Analysis	
Survival	Variables	HR	p	HR Cox Regression	p
Overall Survival	-PCI	1.15 (1.10–1.20)	0.000	1.139 (1.089–1.192)	**0.001**
	-Neoadjuvant Chemo	1.93 (1.16–3.21)	0.012		
	-CC score	7.67 (2.25–26.18)	0.001		
	-Operative time	0.48 (0.10–2.34)	0.002		
	-Severe complications (III–IV) *	1.32 (1.05–1.65)	0.016		
	-Transfusion	1.78 (1.07–2.96)	0.0927		
Disease Free Survival	-PCI	1.09 (1.05–1.13)	0.000	1.087 (1.047–1.128)	**0.001**
	-Neoadjuvant Chemo	1.82 (1.18–2.82)	0.007	1.738 (1.092–2.765)	**0.020**
	-No. of liver metastases	25.51 (3.11–209.4)	0.003		
	-Operative time	1.00 (1.00–1.00)	0.029		
	-Severe complications (III–IV) *	25.51 (1.04–1.50)	0.016		
	-Native KRAS	9.70 (1.01–93.23)	0.049		

* III–IV Clavien–Dindo complications.

4. Discussion

Peritoneal and liver metastases are the two most frequent causes of death in colorectal cancer [10]. In addition, peritoneal dissemination is the one with the worst prognosis with a 30% lower survival, probably due to a lower response to systemic chemotherapy [4,29], or as recently described, by the possibility of representing a mesenchymal molecular subtype (CMS4) with a strong TGF-activation, immune suppression and stromal invasion [30]. Furthermore, it is estimated that approximately 8% of patients with colon cancer develop hepatic and peritoneal metastases simultaneously [1,7] and until recently, these patients were considered unresectable and only amenable to palliative adjuvant chemotherapy with an overall survival of 12 months [4,7]. Indeed, the De Cuba meta-analysis reflected that as much as 25% of scheduled patients for liver surgery were discarded due to the finding of peritoneal metastases [31]. Elias et al. and a consensus statement has shown that patients with up to three liver metastases and a low peritoneal tumor burden (PCI < 12) did not suppose an absolute contraindication for a simultaneous treatment with CRC-HIPEC [9,10,32,33]. Following these criteria and after obtaining a complete tumor resection, a median OS of 25–45 months and an acceptable morbidity and mortality rates could be achieved [1,16,32,34]. In a previous report, we updated our results and showed a median OS of 44 months in patients with simultaneous peritoneal and liver metastases resection [17].

4.1. Morbidity and Mortality

Although several studies have reported acceptable results in selected patients treated with simultaneous resection, its general application still remains controversial due to the increased morbidity, mortality, and delayed administration of adjuvant chemotherapy [1,2,9–19,22,33,34]. One added difficulty for this simultaneous approach is the different intraoperative management (restriction of intravenous fluids required during liver resection versus an increased volume perfusion administered during peritoneal cytoreduction and HIPEC) [1]. In this sense, actual goal-guided fluid therapy has helped to treat this problem [23]. The results of this study showed that patients in the LR+ group presented more postoperative complications and longer ICU and hospital stays, despite having a PCI less than 12 and ≤3 liver metastases, which fulfils the criteria proposed by Elias and other authors [9–11]. Severe Clavien–Dindo complications were 19.5% vs. 40.5% in LR− and LR+, respectively (p: 0.017), and these results are consistent with those found in the literature, which reflects the greater complexity of these interventions, with longer operative time and higher PCI ranging from 15 to 50% [9,11,16,20,21,31,35,36]. In fact, liver metastases and perioperative transfusion were predictors of serious complications in the multivariate analysis (Table 5). Maggiori et al. [34] demonstrated greater postoperative morbidity only in patients with a PCI > 12 who underwent major hepatectomy, considering this association as a limitation factor for the simultaneous approach. Interestingly, this same author and Navez et al. [14] did not related such morbidity to the liver resection. Other authors like Saxena et al. [37] and El-Nakeep et al. [35], did not find significant differences in severe morbidity. The most frequent serious complication in our study was nosocomial pneumonia (23 patients). Eight patients developed respiratory distress and two of them died for this reason. These results force us to insist on activating preventive measures with preoperative and postoperative respiratory physiotherapy, as well as promoting early extubation and mobilization [38]. Intraabdominal abscesses were also significantly more frequent in the LR+ group and this finding may be explained by the fact that in as many as 62.5% of the cases, the infected collection was in the hepatectomy bed. This has been also described by other authors [1]. Unlike severe morbidity, ninety-days mortality has experienced a significant decrease, with figures around 4%, due to better patient selection and postoperative management [1,2,11,39] Our results are in that range and did not show significant differences between the two groups.

4.2. Survival and Recurrence

Recently, OS has been increased with the administration of oxaliplatin and irinotecan and the addition of targeted therapies (e.g., bevacizumab and cetuximab) in patients with metastatic colon cancer [40]. However, the survival analysis has biases that are difficult to avoid in patients who are candidates for simultaneous liver and peritoneal cytoreduction surgery because there are no randomized studies that compare the survival obtained with chemotherapy alone [31,34,41]. Although the PRODIGE 7 trial raised questions regarding the efficacy of HIPEC with oxaliplatine [42] in peritoneal metastases, such long-term outcomes (median survival of 42 months and 5-year survival of 40%) have never been published before [42,43]. Our results in the LR+ group (OS and DFS of 43 and 11.7 months, respectively,) are in accordance with those described in previous publications, which range from 15 to 47 months in OS and 8.5 to 25 in DFS, in selected patients (PCI < 12, ≤3 liver metastasis and complete cytoreduction) with concurrent liver and peritoneal metastasis [2,10,11,16,44]. PCI and CC Score are considered the most important prognostic factors in patients with CP [11,45] and a threshold of 17 PCI points has been described as limit for resectability in peritoneal carcinomatosis of colorectal origin [46]. Although the univariate analysis showed differences in the overall survival for the CC score, duration of surgery, serious complications and transfusion, PCI was the only predictive factor for OS

(HR: 1.139 (1.089–1.192) $p < 0.001$). However, PCI and neoadjuvant chemotherapy were also predictive factors for DFS (HR: 1.087 (1.047–1.128) $p < 0.001$) and (HR: 1.738 (1.092–2.765) p: 0.020). For now, we do not have a clear explanation for this last result. One hypothesis could be that those patients who receive neoadjuvant chemotherapy had a higher tumor burden. Despite the radical nature of the surgery, 75% of the patients had a recurrence during the follow-up period. The recurrence rate was similar in both groups, but as described by other authors, the LR+ group had a significant higher liver recurrence (p: 0.049) [11,44].

Limitations of this study are the retrospectively nature, the relatively small sample size of the LR+ group and the strict criteria for patient selection. Another limitation is the use of different intraperitoneal cytostatics, but this heterogeneity reflects the evolution of HIPEC treatment over time.

In conclusion, simultaneous peritoneal and liver resection is associated with increased postoperative morbidity and hospital stay, but with similar postoperative mortality and OS and disease-free survival. These results reflect the evolution of these patients considered inoperable until recently and justify the trend to incorporate this surgical strategy within a multimodal therapeutic plan in highly selected patient.

Author Contributions: Conceptualization: R.M.-S., J.J.S.-S., C.P.-F. and J.C.R.-P.; Methodology: R.M.-S. and J.J.S.-S.; Validation: J.M.M.-C., F.J.M.-R., E.P.-Z., F.X.G.-A., M.G.-M. and S.G.; Investigation: C.P.-F. and J.C.R.-P.; Data curation: J.L.-M. Resources: M.A.-M. and M.A.O.; Writing: R.M.-S. and J.J.S.-S.; Supervision: R.M.-S., J.J.S.-S., C.P.-F. and F.X.G.-A. All authors have read and agreed to the published version of the manuscript.

Funding: This research was coordinated by ProA Capital, Halekulani S.L., MJR. It was co-financed by the European Development Regional Fund, 'A way to achieve Europe', as well as P2022/BMD-7321 (Community of Madrid, Spain).

Institutional Review Board Statement: This study was approved by the Institutional Review Board Statement of Universitary Hospital of Son Espases, Palma Mallorca, Spain with the number 727-23.

Informed Consent Statement: Informed consent was obtained from all subjects involved in the study.

Data Availability Statement: The data of the study were extracted from a prospective database in which the anonymity of the patients was sought.

Acknowledgments: Our thanks to AR Millán Pons from the Methodological and Statistical Support Platform of the Balearic Islands Health Research Institute. Palma de Mallorca. Spain.

Conflicts of Interest: The authors declare no conflict of interest.

References

1. Cloyd, J.M.; Abdel-Misih, S.; Hays, J.; Dillhoff, M.E.; Pawlik, T.M.; Schmidt, C. Impact of Synchronous Liver Resection on the Perioperative Outcomes of Patients Undergoing CRS-HIPEC. *J. Gastrointest. Surg.* **2018**, *22*, 1576–1584. [CrossRef] [PubMed]
2. Downs-Canner, S.; Shuai, Y.; Ramalingam, L.; Pingpank, J.F.; Holtzman, M.P.; Zeh, H.J.; Bartlett, D.L.; Choudry, H.A. Safety and efficacy of combined resection of colorectal peritoneal and liver metastases. *J. Surg. Res.* **2017**, *219*, 194–201. [CrossRef] [PubMed]
3. Hadden, W.J.; De Reuver, P.R.; Brown, K.; Mittal, A.; Samra, J.S.; Hugh, T.J. Resection of colorectal liver metastases and extra-hepatic disease: A systematic review and proportional meta- analysis of survival outcomes. *Int. Hepato-Pancreato-Biliary Assoc.* **2016**, *18*, 209–220. [CrossRef]
4. Franko, J.; Shi, Q.; Meyers, J. Prognosis of colorectal peritoneal metastases: An analysis of 10,553 patients treated with systemic therapy in prospective randomized trials (ARCAD database) of individual patient data from prospective randomised trials from the Analysis and Research in C. *Lancet Oncol.* **2016**, *17*, 1709–1719. [CrossRef]
5. Cao, C.Q.; Yan, T.D.; Liauw, W.; Morris, D.L. Comparison of Optimally Resected Hepatectomy and Peritonectomy Patients With Colorectal Cancer Metastasis. *J. Surg. Oncol.* **2009**, *100*, 529–533. [CrossRef] [PubMed]
6. Blackham, A.U.; Russell, G.B.; Stewart IV, J.H.; Votanopoulos, K.; Levine, E.A.; Shen, P. Metastatic colorectal cancer: Survival comparison of hepatic resection versus cytoreductive surgery and hyperthermic intraperitoneal chemotherapy. *Ann. Surg. Oncol.* **2014**, *21*, 2667–2674. [CrossRef]
7. Thomassen, I.; van Gestel, Y.R.; Lemmens, V.E.; de Hingh, I.H. Incidence, Prognosis, and Treatment Options for Patients With Synchronous Peritoneal Carcinomatosis and Liver Metastases from Colorectal Origin. *Dis. Colon Rectum* **2013**, *56*, 1373–1380. [CrossRef]

8. Shubert, C.R.; Habermann, E.B.; Bergquist, J.R.; Thiels, C.A.; Thomsen, K.M.; Kremers, W.K.; Kendrick, M.L.; Cima, R.R.; Nagorney, D.M. A NSQIP Review of Major Morbidity and Mortality of Synchronous Liver Resection for Colorectal Metastasis Stratified by Extent of Liver Resection and Type of Colorectal Resection. *J. Gastrointest. Surg.* **2015**, *19*, 1982–1994. [CrossRef]
9. Elias, D.; Benizri, E.; Pocard, M.; Ducreux, M.; Boige, V.; Lasser, P. Treatment of synchronous peritoneal carcinomatosis and liver metastases from colorectal cancer. *Eur. J. Surg. Oncol.* **2006**, *32*, 632–636. [CrossRef]
10. Alzahrani, N.; Ung, L.; Valle, S.J.; Liauw, W.; Morris, D.L. Synchronous liver resection with cytoreductive surgery for the treatment of liver and peritoneal metastases from colon cancer: Results from an Australian centre. *ANZ J. Surg.* **2015**, *87*, E167–E172. [CrossRef]
11. Lo Dico, R.; Faron, M.; Yonemura, Y.; Glehen, O.; Pocard, M.; Sardi, A.; Hübner, M.; Baratti, D.; Liberale, G.; Kartheuser, A.; et al. Combined liver resection and cytoreductive surgery with HIPEC for metastatic colorectal cancer: Results of a worldwide analysis of 565 patients from the Peritoneal Surface Oncology Group International (PSOGI). *Eur. J. Surg. Oncol.* **2021**, *47*, 89–100. [CrossRef] [PubMed]
12. Kianmanesh, R.; Scaringi, S.; Sabate, J.-M.; Castel, B.; Pons-Kerjean, N.; Coffin, B.; Hay, J.-M.; Flamant, Y.; Msika, S. Iterative Cytoreductive Surgery Associated With Hyperthermic Intraperitoneal Chemotherapy for Treatment of Peritoneal Carcinomatosis of Colorectal Origin With or Without Liver Metastases. *Ann. Surg.* **2007**, *245*, 597–603. [CrossRef] [PubMed]
13. Delhorme, J.B.; Dupont-Kazma, L.; Addeo, P.; Lefebvre, F.; Triki, E.; Romain, B.; Meyer, N.; Bachellier, P.; Rohr, S.; Brigand, C. Peritoneal carcinomatosis with synchronous liver metastases from colorectal cancer: Who will benefit from complete cytoreductive surgery? *Int. J. Surg.* **2016**, *25*, 98–105. [CrossRef] [PubMed]
14. Navez, J.; Remue, C.; Leonard, D.; Bachmann, R.; Kartheuser, A.; Hubert, C.; Coubeau, L.; Komuta, M.; Van den Eynde, M.; Zech, F.; et al. Surgical Treatment of Colorectal Cancer with Peritoneal and Liver Metastases Using Combined Liver and Cytoreductive Surgery and Hyperthermic Intraperitoneal Chemotherapy: Report from a Single-Centre Experience. *Ann. Surg. Oncol.* **2016**, *23*, 666–673. [CrossRef]
15. Mouw, T.J.; Lu, J.; Woody-Fowler, M.; Ashcraft, J.; Valentino, J.; DiPasco, P.; Mammen, J.; Al-Kasspooles, M. Morbidity and mortality of synchronous hepatectomy with cytoreductive surgery/hyperthermic intraperitoneal chemotherapy (CRS/HIPEC). *J. Gastrointest. Oncol.* **2018**, *9*, 828–832. [CrossRef]
16. Flood, M.P.; Das Atalindra, A.; Soucisse, M.L.; Kong, J.; Ramsay, R.G.; Michael, M.; Hons, M.B.B.S.; Hons, B.S.; Loveday, B.P.T.; Warrier, S.K. Synchronous Liver Resection, Cytoreductive Surgery, and Hyperthermic Intraperitoneal Chemotherapy for Colorectal Liver and Peritoneal Metastases: A Systematic Review and Meta-analysis. *Dis. Colon Rectum* **2021**, *64*, 754–764. [CrossRef]
17. Morales Soriano, R.; Morón Canis, J.M.; Molina Romero, X.; Pérez Celada, J.; Tejada Gavela, S.; Segura Sampedro, J.J.; Jiménez Morillas, P.; Díaz Jover, P.; García Pérez, J.M.; Sena Ruiz, F.; et al. Influence of simultaneous liver and peritoneal resection on postoperative morbi-mortality and survival in patients with colon cancer treated with surgical cytoreduction and intraperitoneal hyperthermic chemotherapy. *Cirugía Española* **2017**, *95*, 214–221. [CrossRef]
18. Chua, T.C.; Yan, T.D.; Zhao, J.; Morris, D.L. Peritoneal carcinomatosis and liver metastases from colorectal cancer treated with cytoreductive surgery perioperative intraperitoneal chemotherapy and liver resection. *Eur. J. Surg. Oncol.* **2009**, *35*, 1299–1305. [CrossRef]
19. Allard, M.A.; Adam, R.; Ruiz, A.; Vibert, E.; Paule, B.; Levi, F.; Sebagh, M.; Guettier, C.; Azoulay, D.; Castaing, D. Is unexpected peritoneal carcinomatosis still a contraindication for resection of colorectal liver metastases?: Combined resection of colorectal liver metastases with peritoneal deposits discovered intra-operatively. *Eur. J. Surg. Oncol.* **2013**, *39*, 981–987. [CrossRef]
20. Soldevila-Verdeguer, C.; Segura-Sampedro, J.J.; Pineño-Flores, C.; Sanchís-Cortés, P.; González-Argente, X.; Morales-Soriano, R. Hepatic resection and blood transfusion increase morbidity after cytoreductive surgery and HIPEC for colorectal carcinomatosis. *Clin. Transl. Oncol.* **2020**, *22*, 2032–2039. [CrossRef]
21. Chua, T.C.; Yan, T.D.; Saxena, A.; Morris, D.L. Should the treatment of peritoneal carcinomatosis by cytoreductive surgery and hyperthermic intraperitoneal chemotherapy still be regarded as a highly morbid procedure? A systematic review of morbidity and mortality. *Ann. Surg.* **2009**, *249*, 900–907. [CrossRef] [PubMed]
22. Segura-Sampedro, J.J.; Morales-Soriano, R.; Pineño Flores, C.; Craus-Miguel, A.; Sugarbaker, P.H. Laparoscopy technique in the setting of peritoneal metastases to avoid port site relapse. *Surg. Oncol.* **2021**, *37*, 15–18. [CrossRef] [PubMed]
23. Esteve-Pérez, N.; Ferrer-Robles, A.; Gómez-Romero, G.; Fabián-Gonzalez, D.; Verd-Rodriguez, M.; Mora-Fernandez, L.C.; Segura-Sampedro, J.J.; Tejada-Gavela, S.; Morales-Soriano, R. Goal-directed therapy in cytoreductive surgery with hyperthermic intraperitoneal chemotherapy: A prospective observational study. *Clin. Transl. Oncol.* **2019**, *21*, 451–458. [CrossRef] [PubMed]
24. Yonemura, Y.; Bandou, E.; Kawamura, T.; Endou, Y.; Sasaki, T. Quantitative prognostic indicators of peritoneal dissemination of gastric cancer. *Eur. J. Surg. Oncol.* **2006**, *32*, 602–606. [CrossRef] [PubMed]
25. Esquivel, J.; Sticca, R.; Sugarbaker, P.; Levine, E.; Yan, T.D.; Alexander, R.; Baratti, D.; Bartlett, D.; Barone, R.; Barrios, P.; et al. Cytoreductive Surgery and Hyperthermic Intraperitoneal Chemotherapy in the Management of Peritoneal Surface Malignancies of Colonic Origin: A Consensus Statement. *Ann. Surg. Oncol.* **2007**, *14*, 128–133. [CrossRef]
26. González-Bayón, L.; González-Moreno, S.; Ortega-Pérez, G. Safety considerations for operating room personnel during hyperthermic intraoperative intraperitoneal chemotherapy perfusion. *Eur. J. Surg. Oncol.* **2006**, *32*, 619–624. [CrossRef]
27. González-Moreno, S.; González-Bayón, L.; Ortega-Pérez, G. Hyperthermic Intraperitoneal Chemotherapy. Methodology and Safety Considerations. *Surg. Oncol. Clin. North Am.* **2012**, *21*, 543–557. [CrossRef]
28. Clavien, P.A.; Barkun, J.; De Oliveira, M.L.; Vauthey, J.N.; Dindo, D.; Schulick, R.D.; De Santibañes, E.; Pekolj, J.; Slankamenac, K.; Bassi, C.; et al. The clavien-dindo classification of surgical complications: Five-year experience. *Ann. Surg.* **2009**, *250*, 187–196. [CrossRef]

29. Franko, J.; Shi, Q.; Goldman, C.D.; Pockaj, B.A.; Nelson, G.D.; Goldberg, R.M.; Pitot, H.C.; Grothey, A.; Alberts, S.R.; Sargent, D.J. Treatment of colorectal peritoneal carcinomatosis with systemic chemotherapy: A pooled analysis of North Central Cancer Treatment Group phase III trials N9741 and N9841. *J. Clin. Oncol.* **2012**, *30*, 263–267. [CrossRef]
30. Lenos, K.J.; Bach, S.; Ferreira Moreno, L.; ten Hoorn, S.; Sluiter, N.R.; Bootsma, S.; Vieira Braga, F.A.; Nijman, L.E.; van den Bosch, T.; Miedema, D.M.; et al. Molecular characterization of colorectal cancer related peritoneal metastatic disease. *Nat. Commun.* **2022**, *13*, 4443. [CrossRef]
31. de Cuba, E.M.V.; Kwakman, R.; Knol, D.L.; Bonjer, H.J.; Meijer, G.A.; te Velde, E.A. Cytoreductive surgery and HIPEC for peritoneal metastases combined with curative treatment of colorectal liver metastases. Systematic review of all literature and meta-analysis of observational studies. *Cancer Treat. Rev.* **2013**, *39*, 321–327. [CrossRef] [PubMed]
32. Elias, D.; Dube, P.; Bonvalot, S.; Meshaka, P.; Manai, M.; Cavalcanti, A.; Lasser, P. Treatment of liver metastases with moderate peritoneal carcinomatosis by hepatectomy and cytoreductive surgery follow by inmediate post-operative intraperitoneal chemotherapy: Feasibility and preliminary results. *Hepato-Gastroenterol.* **1999**, *46*, 360–363. [PubMed]
33. Esquivel, J.; Elias, D.; Baratti, D.; Kusamura, S.; Deraco, M. Consensus statement on the loco regional treatment of colorectal cancer with peritoneal dissemination. *J. Surg. Oncol.* **2008**, *98*, 263–267. [CrossRef]
34. Maggiori, L.; Goéré, D.; Viana, B.; Tzanis, D.; Dumont, F.; Honoré, C.; Eveno, C.; Elias, D. Should Patients With Peritoneal Carcinomatosis of Colorectal Origin With Synchronous Liver Metastases Be Treated With a Curative Intent? A Case-Control Study. *Ann. Surg.* **2013**, *258*, 116–121. [CrossRef] [PubMed]
35. El-Nakeep, S.; Rashad, N.; Oweira, H.; Schmidt, J.; Helbling, D.; Giryes, A.; Petrausch, U.; Mehrabi, A.; Decker, M.; Abdel-Rahman, O. Intraperitoneal chemotherapy and cytoreductive surgery for peritoneal metastases coupled with curative treatment of colorectal liver metastases: An updated systematic review. *Expert Rev. Gastroenterol. Hepatol.* **2017**, *11*, 249–258. [CrossRef] [PubMed]
36. Maggiori, L.; Elias, D. Curative treatment of colorectal peritoneal carcinomatosis: Current status and future trends. *Eur. J. Surg. Oncol.* **2010**, *36*, 599–603. [CrossRef] [PubMed]
37. Saxena, A.; Valle, S.J.; Liauw, W.; Morris, D.L. Limited synchronous hepatic resection does not compromise peri-operative outcomes or survival after cytoreductive surgery and hyperthermic intraperitoneal chemotherapy. *J. Surg. Oncol.* **2017**, *115*, 417–424. [CrossRef]
38. Hübner, M.; Kusamura, S.; Villeneuve, L.; Al-niaimi, A.; Alyami, M.; Balonov, K.; Bell, J.; Bristow, R.; Glehen, O.; Fagotti, A.; et al. European Journal of Surgical Oncology Guidelines for Perioperative Care in Cytoreductive Surgery (CRS) with or without hyperthermic IntraPEritoneal chemotherapy (HIPEC): Enhanced recovery after surgery (ERAS®) Society Recommendations d Part I: Pre. *Eur. J. Surg. Oncol.* **2020**, *46*, 2292–2310. [CrossRef]
39. Saxena, A.; Yan, T.D.; Chua, T.C.; Morris, D.L. Critical assessment of risk factors for complications after cytoreductive surgery and perioperative intraperitoneal chemotherapy for pseudomyxoma peritonei. *Ann. Surg. Oncol.* **2010**, *17*, 1291–1301. [CrossRef]
40. Loupakis, F.; Cremolini, C.; Masi, G.; Lonardi, S.; Zagonel, V.; Salvatore, L.; Cortesi, E.; Tomasello, G.; Ronzoni, M.; Spadi, R.; et al. Initial Therapy with FOLFOXIRI and Bevacizumab for Metastatic Colorectal Cancer. *N. Engl. J. Med.* **2014**, *371*, 1609–1618. [CrossRef]
41. Pinto, A.; Hobeika, C.; Philis, A.; Kirzin, S.; Carrère, N.; Ghouti, L. Synchronous liver metastases and peritoneal carcinomatosis from colorectal cancer: Different strategies for curative treatment? *Langenbeck's Arch. Surg.* **2019**, *404*, 477–488. [CrossRef] [PubMed]
42. Quénet, F.; Elias, D.; Roca, L.; Goéré, D.; Ghouti, L.; Pocard, M.; Facy, O.; Arvieux, C.; Lorimier, G. Cytoreductive surgery plus hyperthermic intraperitoneal chemotherapy versus cytoreductive surgery alone for colorectal peritoneal metastases (PRODIGE 7): A multicentre, randomised, open-label, phase 3 trial. *Lancet Oncol.* **2021**, *22*, 256–266. [CrossRef] [PubMed]
43. Elias, D.; Lefevre, J.H.; Chevalier, J.; Brouquet, A.; Marchal, F.; Classe, J.M.; Ferron, G.; Guilloit, J.M.; Meeus, P.; Goéré, D.; et al. Complete cytoreductive surgery plus intraperitoneal chemohyperthermia with oxaliplatin for peritoneal carcinomatosis of colorectal origin. *J. Clin. Oncol.* **2009**, *27*, 681–685. [CrossRef] [PubMed]
44. Lorimier, G.; Linot, B.; Paillocher, N.; Dupoiron, D.; Verrièle, V.; Wernert, R.; Hamy, A.; Capitain, O. Curative cytoreductive surgery followed by hyperthermic intraperitoneal chemotherapy in patients with peritoneal carcinomatosis and synchronous resectable liver metastases arising from colorectal cancer. *Eur. J. Surg. Oncol.* **2017**, *43*, 150–158. [CrossRef] [PubMed]
45. Elias, D.; Faron, M.; Goéré, D.; Dumont, F.; Honoré, C.; Boige, V.; Malka, D.; Ducreux, M. A simple tumor load-based nomogram for surgery in patients with colorectal liver and peritoneal metastases. *Ann. Surg. Oncol.* **2014**, *21*, 2052–2058. [CrossRef]
46. Goéré, D.; Souadka, A.; Faron, M.; Cloutier, A.S.; Viana, B.; Honoré, C.; Dumont, F.; Elias, D. Extent of Colorectal Peritoneal Carcinomatosis: Attempt to Define a Threshold Above Which HIPEC Does Not Offer Survival Benefit: A Comparative Study. *Ann. Surg. Oncol.* **2015**, *22*, 2958–2964. [CrossRef]

Journal of
Clinical Medicine

Article

Under the Hood: Understanding the Features of Mucin in Pseudomyxoma Peritonei

Pedro Villarejo-Campos [1,2,*], Mariano García-Arranz [2,3], Siyuan Qian [1], Santos Jiménez de los Galanes [1], Víctor Domínguez-Prieto [1], Juan Felipe Vélez-Pinto [1], Ismael Guijo Castellano [1], Montiel Jiménez-Fuertes [1], Héctor Guadalajara [1,2] and Damián García-Olmo [1,2,3]

[1] Department of Surgery, Fundación Jiménez Díaz University Hospital, Avda. Reyes Católicos, 2, 28040 Madrid, Spain; siyuan.qianv@quironsalud.es (S.Q.); santos.jimenez@quironsalud.es (S.J.d.l.G.); victor.dominguez@quironsalud.es (V.D.-P.); felipevelezpinto@gmail.com (J.F.V.-P.); iguijo@fjd.es (I.G.C.); montiel.jimenez@quironsalud.es (M.J.-F.); hector.guadalajara@uam.es (H.G.); damian.garcia@uam.es (D.G.-O.)

[2] Department of Surgery, Universidad Autónoma de Madrid, C/Arzobispo Morcillo s/n, 28034 Madrid, Spain; mariano.garcia@quironsalud.es

[3] New Therapies Laboratory, Health Research Institute-Fundación Jiménez Díaz University Hospital (IIS-FJD), Avda. Reyes Católicos, 2, 28040 Madrid, Spain

* Correspondence: pedro.villarejo@quironsalud.es

Abstract: Pseudomyxoma peritonei (PMP) is a rare malignant growth characterized by the production of mucin and the potential for peritoneal relapse. This study aimed to investigate the immunohistochemical and biological characteristics of mucin in patients with cellular and acellular PMP. We prospectively analyzed mucin specimens obtained from our patient cohort and described the composition and type of mucin present in each sample. A metagenomic analysis of the samples was performed to investigate the bacterial composition of the PMP microbiome. Secreted mucins 2 and 5AC and membrane-associated mucin-1 were the primary components of mucin in both cellular and acellular tumor specimens. The metagenomic study revealed a predominance of the phylum *Proteobacteria* and the genus *Pseudomonas*. Notably, *Pseudomonas plecoglossicida*, a species not previously reported in the human microbiome, was found to be the most abundant organism in the mucin of pseudomyxoma peritonei. Our findings suggest that the presence of MUC-2 and mucin colonization by Pseudomonas are characteristic features of both cellular and acellular disease. These results may have significant implications for the diagnosis and treatment of this rare entity.

Keywords: pseudomyxoma peritonei; mucin; MUC-2; microbiome; pseudomonas

1. Introduction

Pseudomyxoma peritonei (PMP) is a rare syndrome characterized by the buildup of mucin in the peritoneal cavity, often resulting from ruptured appendiceal mucinous neoplasms. While ovarian involvement is common in this condition, it is usually metastatic in nature [1]. Ovarian cystic teratoma is the only tumor of ovarian origin identified as a likely cause of PMP. Although less common, gastrointestinal mucinous adenocarcinomas and urachal cancer have also been identified as potential origins of PMP [2].

According to the Peritoneal Surface Oncology Group International (PSOGI) classification, acellular mucin is characterized by an absence of tumor epithelial cells. In contrast, PMP containing neoplastic epithelial cells in the mucin can be classified into three types based on histopathologic features and the volume of tumor cells [3]:

- Low-grade mucinous carcinoma peritonei: characterized by low-grade cytology, few mitoses, and scant mucinous tumor epithelium (<20% of tumor volume).
- High-grade mucinous carcinoma peritonei is characterized by the presence of at least one of the following features: high-grade cytology, infiltration of adjacent tissues,

invasion of vascular lymphatic vessels or surrounding nerves, cribriform growth, or extensive mucinous tumor epithelium (>20% of tumor volume).

- High-grade mucinous carcinoma peritonei with signet ring cells: characterized by the presence of neoplastic signet ring cells (signet ring cells $\geq$ 10%).

Furthermore, the Ki-67 proliferation index has recently been proposed as a tool for stratifying high-grade PMP and predicting prognosis [4].

While the classification and prognosis of patients with PMP depends on the aforementioned histopathologic features, mucin itself has unique characteristics that warrant further study. Despite the current treatment option of cytoreductive surgery and hyperthermic intraperitoneal chemotherapy (HIPEC) [3,5], tumor recurrence and progression are frequent, with high mortality rates [5]. Therefore, identifying new therapeutic targets is crucial.

Our research aims to investigate the proteomic and biological characteristics of mucinous material in PMP as well as its metagenomic features (i.e., microbiome). We believe that a fuller understanding of mucin may provide insight into the development and progression of the disease, potentially leading to new treatment options for patients.

2. Materials and Methods

Patients: We obtained mucin samples from patients diagnosed with PMP who underwent surgery at Fundación Jiménez Díaz University Hospital from April 2016 to July 2020. All patients received information on the study and provided written consent to participate. The study protocol was approved by the Ethics Committee for Clinical Research of Fundación Jiménez Díaz University Hospital (PIC 75/2016_FJD). The animal study protocol was approved by the Committee on Animal Ethics and Welfare of the Fundación Jiménez Díaz University Hospital Research Institute (PIC 63/2016_FJD). We proposed a pilot study comprising a sample of nine patients who underwent surgical cytoreduction combined with HIPEC. In eight cases, the origin of the PMP was a low-grade appendiceal mucinous neoplasm (LAMN), while in one case a mucinous adenocarcinoma of the colon was the source. Following the postoperative histopathologic study, five of the PMP cases were diagnosed as acellular pseudomyxoma, and four were diagnosed as low-grade peritoneal mucinous carcinoma. In most of the patients included in our study, PMP originated from a perforated LAMN. Patients who underwent successful complete cytoreduction have remained alive without relapse. However, there was one patient who had incomplete cytoreduction. Unfortunately, this patient relapsed 6 months after the incomplete cytoreduction and eventually died within 17 months (Table 1).

Table 1. Clinical and histological features.

Age	Sex	Primary Tumor	Perforated	PMP Classification	Preoperative Chemotherapy	Cytoreduction Score	Current Status	Overall Survival (Months)
59	♂	LAMN	Yes	Metachronous LMCP (LMCP-1)	No	CC0	AWR	84
44	♀	LAMN	Yes	Synchronous AM (AM-1)	No	CC0	AWR	79
45	♂	LAMN	Yes	Metachronous AM (AM-2)	No	CC0	AWR	75
75	♀	LAMN	Yes	Metachronous AM (AM-3)	No	CC0	AWR	72
73	♀	MCA	No	Metachronous LMCP (LMCP-2)	No	CC0	AWR	54
80	♀	LAMN	No	Synchronous LMCP (LMCP-3)	No	CC1	DWR	17

Low-grade appendiceal mucinous neoplasm (LAMN). Mucinous colonic adenocarcinoma (MCA). Low-grade mucinous carcinoma peritonei (LMCP). Acellular mucin (AM). CC0: completed cytoreduction. CC1: residual tumor nodules < 0.25 cm. Alive without recurrence (AWR). Dead with recurrence (DWR).

Subsequently, all histopathologic analyses were repeated to detect neoplastic cells in mucin samples. Six consecutive patients were included in the final sample: three with acellular mucin and three with neoplastic cells in the mucin. The multi-step process followed to characterize mucin is described below.

Mucin degradation: The viscosity of the mucinous component in PMP is related to such characteristics of mucin as protein concentration or cellularity (higher cellularity and protein concentration, greater sclerosis) and other external factors related to the microenvironment such as hyperosmolarity, pH < 4, or the existence of trefoil factors (soluble peptides secreted by goblet cells of the digestive tract that promote mucin viscosity) [6]. Mucolytics such as bromelain and N-acetylcysteine can be used to digest both soft and hard mucin (Figure 1) [7,8]. Soft mucin is easily degradable, while hard mucin exhibits greater sclerosis and an increased resistance to degradation [7].

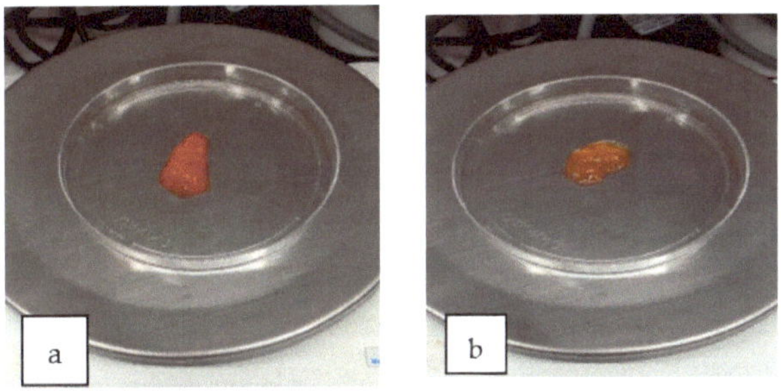

Figure 1. (**a**) Hard mucin; (**b**) soft mucin.

Soft mucin was digested with a solution consisting of 0.3 mg/mL bromelain and 2% N-acetylcysteine and left to incubate for 90–120 min at 37 °C. Hard mucin required a longer incubation time to degrade (≤240 min).

Proteomic analysis: Following mucin digestion with bromelain and N-acetylcysteine, proteins were extracted using RIPA lysis buffer (Tris-HCl (50 nM), NaCl (150 mM), EDTA (1 mM), Nonidet P-40 (1%), DOC (0.5%), and SDS (80.1%)). The proteins were then quantified by Coomassie Brilliant blue R-250, running the gel at 100 V for 1.15 h. Finally, 20 μL per well was loaded into a precast gel (Mini-Protean TGx 4–15%, Bio-Rad, Hercules, CA, USA) using 4× Laemmli sample buffer (Bio-Rad, Hercules, CA, USA) and 5% β-mercaptoethanol as loading buffer, according to manufacturer recommendations. Subsequently, each membrane was incubated overnight with specific antibodies against the different mucins: MUC-1 (Proteintech/Fisher Scientific, Madrid, Spain), MUC-2 (ABCore Ramona-San Diego County, CA, USA), MUC-3 (Santa Cruz Biotechnology, Heidelberg, Germany), MUC-5AC (Cloud-Clone Corp/Biogen Científica, Madrid, Spain), MUC-13 (Santa Cruz Biotechnology, Heidelberg, Germany), and MUC-16 (Santa Cruz, Biotechnology, Heidelberg, Germany) at 4 °C and washed 4× with TTBS under gentle agitation for 15 min; goat anti-mouse secondary antibody (Southern Biotech/Bionova, Madrid, Spain) was added (MUC 2, 3, 13, and 16) as well as goat anti-rabbit (Southern Biotech) (MUC 1, 5AC), incubating for 1 h at room temperature under agitation. The membranes were washed with TTBS for 15 min and analyzed in an iBright system (Thermo Fisher, Madrid, Spain).

Microbiome analysis: The prokaryotic 16S ribosomal RNA (rRNA) gene is frequently used in metagenomic surveys of microbial populations due to its conserved and variable regions, which facilitate sequencing and phylogenetic classification. The microbiota in human and mouse biospecimens can be effectively studied through targeted amplification of bacterial 16S rRNA genes [9]. To identify the bacteria present in cellular and acellular mucin specimens, we performed 16S gene sequencing on the DNA extracted from these samples. Subsequently, we inoculated the mucin samples into both immunocompetent and immunocompromised mice to study the behavior of the microbiome in these experimental models.

Generation of 16S amplicons and amplicon sequencing was performed using the Illumina Miseq platform in the Genomics Unit of the Madrid Scientific Park. An initial PCR was performed with the Q5® Hot Start High-Fidelity DNA Polymerase enzyme (New England Biolabs, Barcelona, Spain) using 300 pg of DNA. The primers used amplified the V3-V4 region of 16S and add extra sequences on which the second PCR was performed: 5′-ACACTGACGACATGGTTCTACA CCTACGGGNGGCWGCAG-3′ and 5′-TACGGTAGCAGAGACTTGGTCTGACTACHVGG GTATCTAAT CC-3′. Cycling of the first PCR was performed as follows: 1 × 98 °C 30 s; 23 × (98 °C 10 s, 50 °C 20 s, 72 °C 20 s); and 1 × 72 °C 2 min.

We performed a second PCR on the amplification products of the first PCR using the Q5® Hot Start High-Fidelity DNA Polymerase enzyme, with the following primers (5′-AATGATACGGCGACCACCGA GATCTACACTGACGACATGGTTCTACA-3′ and 5′-CAAGCAGAAGACGGCATACGAGAT-[10 nucleotides] -TACGGTAGCAGAGACTTGGTCT-3′) from Fluidigm (Illumina Sequencers, Madrid, Spain). Cycling of this PCR was as follows: 1 × 98 °C 30 s; 14 × (98 °C 10 s, 60 °C 20 s, 72 °C 20 s); and 1 × 72 °C 2 min.

The final products were quantified by Bioanalyzer (Agilent Technologies, Santa Clara, CA, USA) to prepare an equimolecular pool that was subsequently purified by selecting the band of interest in an agarose gel with SYBR Gold (Thermo Fisher). After, the pool of amplicons was quantified by qPCR using the Kapa SYBR FAST qPCR kit for Light Cycler 480 master mix and a reference library belonging to the Genomics Unit of the Madrid Scientific Park.

Finally, the pool of amplicons was sequenced with the Illumina Miseq platform following the manufacturer's instructions, in a paired-end (2 × 300 bp) sequencing run using MiSeq reagent kit v3-600 cycles (Illumina, Eindhoven, The Netherlands).

3. Results

Proteomic analysis revealed the presence of secretory mucins MUC-2 and MUC-5AC, as well as the membrane mucin MUC-1, in all samples analyzed, predominantly MUC-2 (Table 2). We further detected the MUC-1 protein in mucin for the first time (MUC-1 overexpression was previously described only in tumor tissue). No other mucin types were identified, and there were no significant differences in the composition or distribution of mucin types between acellular and cellular samples (Figure 2).

Table 2. Proteomic analysis.

Patients	Samples	Mucin-1 (μg/μL)	Mucin-2 (μg/μL)	Mucin-5AC (μg/μL)
LMCP-1	Cellular mucin	46	82	40
LMCP-2	Cellular mucin	33	77	31
LMCP-3	Cellular mucin	35	70	42
AM-1	Acellular mucin	44	68	40
AM-2	Acellular mucin	44	68	40
AM-3	Acellular mucin	43	75	40

Low-grade mucinous carcinoma peritonei (LMCP). Acellular mucin (AM).

To examine the microbiota in mucin samples, we conducted 16S sequencing and identified different bacterial taxa. The most frequently detected phylum was genomic DNA from *Proteobacteria* in both acellular (82.86%) and cellular (82.52%) mucin, followed by *Actinobacteria* (8.17% and 8.52%, respectively). The most common bacterial order was *Pseudomonadales*, comprising 44.99% of the microbiome in acellular mucin and 44.55% in cellular mucin. The predominant genus was *Pseudomonas*, accounting for about 45% of the germs detected in both mucin groups (Figure 3).

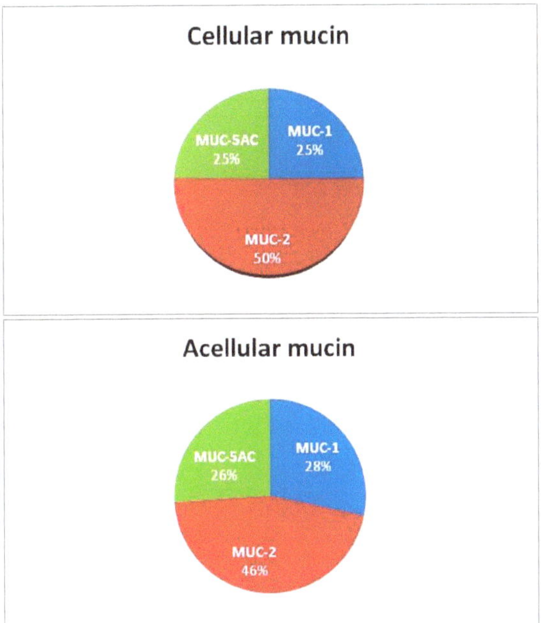

Figure 2. Mucin composition.

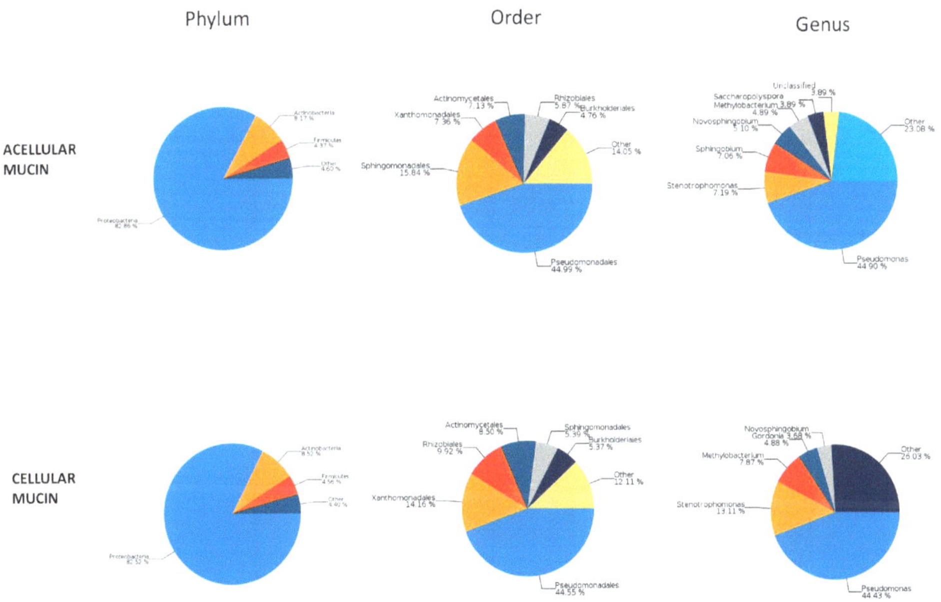

Figure 3. Microbiome analysis.

Interestingly, the microbiota of patients with PMP and acellular mucin was almost identical to that of patients with cellular mucin. This suggests that germ colonization of accumulated mucus in PMP, primarily from *Pseudomonas*, is a specific feature of mucin independent of the patient and tumor histopathology. To confirm this hypothesis, we inoculated mucin samples into immunocompetent (C57) and immunosuppressed (NSG) mice and found that the microbiota was maintained regardless of host species and immune status (Figure 4).

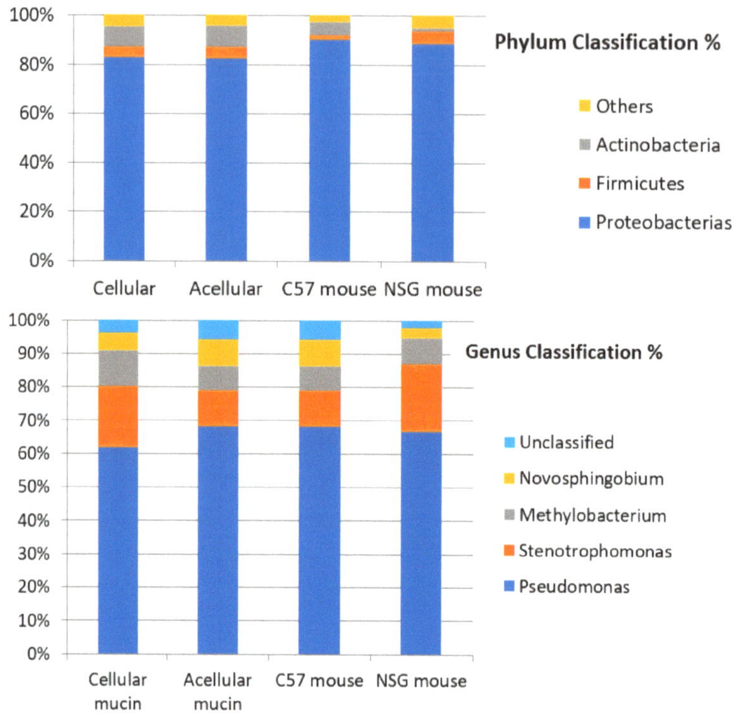

Figure 4. Microbiota of samples collected from patients with PMP and mucin xenoimplants in murine models.

Pseudomonas plecoglossicida was the most frequently identified bacterial species among all the samples analyzed, representing 11–21% of the total bacterial population.

4. Discussion

The overexpression of genes encoding different proteins of the mucin family has been described in the primary and metastatic tumor tissues of PMP. These proteins include mucin-2 (MUC-2), mucin-5AC (MUC-5AC), mucin-5B (MUC-5B), mucin-4 (MUC-4), and mucin-1 (MUC-1) [7,10–17]. The MUC-2, MUC-5AC, and MUC-5B proteins are secreted gel-forming mucins, while the MUC-1 and MUC-4 proteins are membrane-associated mucins [18]. While there is extensive research on the overexpression of mucin in tumor tissues, investigations focusing on mucin itself are considerably more limited (See Table 3 for an overview).

No reports to date have described the protein composition of acellular mucin in PMP. Our results show that the mucus in acellular mucin has a makeup that resembles the mucin of other types of PMP.

Secreted MUC-2 and MUC-5AC are the main components of mucus in PMP. MUC-5AC is expressed in the goblet cells of the gastrointestinal and respiratory epithelium as well as ovarian epithelial cells, whereas MUC-2 expression is specific to goblet cells of the intestinal epithelium [10]. MUC-2 is the only protein that has been consistently described in studies involving PMP, both those performed directly on the protein composition of mucin as well as research using tumor tissues. This pattern of mucin expression explains the appendicular origin of most cases of PMP. MUC-2 is characterized by extensive glycosylation and has been associated with mucus sclerosis and even with patient prognosis in PMP [6].

Table 3. Main research focused on characterizing mucin types in tumor tissue or mucin samples.

	SAMPLES	MUC-2	MUC-5AC	MUC-5B	MUC-1	MUC-6	MUC-4
O'Connell (2002) [7]	Appendix, ovarian, and peritoneal tissues (25)	✓	✓				
Mohamed (2004) [8]	Peritoneal tissue (11)	✓			✓		
Nonaka (2006) [9]	Peritoneal tissue (42)	✓	✓				
Mall (2007) [10]	Mucin (cellular)	✓	✓	✓			✓
Ferreira (2008) [11]	Ovarian tissue (28)	✓			✓		
Baratti (2009) [12]	Peritoneal tissue (85)	✓	✓				
Guo (2011) [13]	Appendix, ovarian, and peritoneal tissues (35)	✓					
Chang (2012) [14]	Appendix tissue (22)	✓	✓				
Pillai (2017) [5]	Mucin (16)	✓	✓	✓			

✓: confirmed finding.

With respect to the microbiome of patients with PMP, it must be noted that the peritoneal cavity is an aseptic anatomical region. Therefore, the bacterial contamination of mucin should originate from the intestine, secondary to the perforation of appendicular mucinous neoplasms [19]. Three identifiable enterotypes have been described in the microbiome of the human gastrointestinal tract, which are defined according to the most prevalent bacterial genera: *Bacteroides* (Enterotype 1), *Prevotella* (Enterotype 2), and *Ruminococcus* (Enterotype 3) [20]. In our study, the predominant bacterial genus in the mucin was *Pseudomonas*. Therefore, we can affirm that it is not a native constituent of the digestive tract microbiome.

Gilbreath et al. [21] were the first to describe the microbiota associated with PMP and to suggest its potential impact on the pathogenesis of this disease. Different methods have been used to study the microbiota of PMP, such as cultures, in situ hybridization, and 16S sequencing. The dominant phylum described is *Proteobacteria*, with a predominance of the *Pseudomonas* genus [19], which coincides with our results.

No previous studies have specifically characterized the microbiota of acellular mucin. The results of the present analysis reveal that it has a microbiota that closely resembles that of other types of PMP. Although the presence of a microbiome having these features is not characteristic of the gastrointestinal tract, it is frequently found in the mucin within the respiratory epithelium of patients with cystic fibrosis disease. Therefore, the existence of abundant mucin and a predominance of *Pseudomonas* in the microbiome are common to PMP and cystic fibrosis. Another shared finding between these two conditions is MUC-2 overexpression, despite the fact that MUC-2 expression is specific to goblet cells of the intestinal epithelium and is not present in the respiratory epithelium under normal conditions [22]. An association between mucus hyperproduction and infection by the genus *Pseudomonas* has been described, as well as a direct relationship between the overexpression of MUC-2 and MUC-5AC and the lipopolysaccharides of this bacterial family [23,24].

Previous studies by our group demonstrated that inoculating acellular mucin in an experimental murine model could be used to reproduce acellular PMP [25]. With these findings in mind, we set out to explore the mechanism by which tumor-cell-free mucin can reproduce and grow. Based on the results of the present research, and taking into account the results of Dohrman A et al. [23] and Ben Mohamed F et al. [24], we can hypothesize that mucin overproduction may be related to colonization by bacteria belonging to the *Pseudomonas* family. To advance our understanding of PMP and improve patient outcomes, future research should investigate the relationship between the mucin microbiome and the aggressiveness and prognosis of the disease.

Findings from this and other research indicate that the microbiota may be a new therapeutic target. Preliminary results from studies that added antibiotics to the standard treatment approach for PMP (i.e., cytoreduction and HIPEC) were inconclusive, although a phase II clinical trial (NCT 02387203) is currently underway to analyze the long-term results of antibiotic administration in patients with PMP [19,26].

Limitations of the study: the primary limitations of this research are the small sample size and the exclusive use of 16S rRNA sequencing for analyzing the microbiome of mucin samples.

No previous publications have described *Pseudomonas plecoglossicida* as the most abundant *Pseudomonas* species in the mucin of PMP. This bacterium has been identified as the cause of hemorrhagic ascites in ayu fish [27], although it has never been found in the human microbiome. We can only speculate whether the occurrence of *Pseudomonas plecoglossicida* is associated with diet or some other cause. It was first identified in diseased ayus (*Plecoglossus altivelis*) [28] and has since been identified in large yellow croakers (*Larimichthys crocea*), groupers (*Epinephelus coioides*), and barramundi (*Lates calcarifer*) [29–32]. These occurrences have been documented solely in fish infections within Asian studies, and there have been no reported cases of their presence in humans. However, it is important to note that this bacterium belongs to the group of *Pseudomonas Putidas*, which are associated with human pathologies, although the transmission mechanism has not been clearly defined [33].

5. Conclusions

Sufficient evidence points to a direct relationship between the dominant microbiome of the pseudomyxoma and the production of mucus in PMP.

Author Contributions: Conceptualization: D.G.-O., M.G.-A. and P.V.-C. Methodology: D.G.-O., M.G.-A., H.G. and P.V.-C. Software: S.Q. Validation: M.G.-A. Investigation: D.G.-O., M.G.-A. and H.G. Resources: S.J.d.l.G., I.G.C., M.J.-F. and S.Q. Data Curation: V.D.-P. and J.F.V.-P. Writing—Original Draft Preparation: P.V.-C., M.G.-A. and D.G.-O. Writing—Review and Eediting: All authors. Funding Acquisition: P.V.-C. and S.J.d.l.G. All authors have read and agreed to the published version of the manuscript.

Funding: This study was funded by grants from the ISCIII-FEDER (Instituto de Salud Carlos III-Fondo Europeo de Desarrollo Regional), Spanish Ministry of Health (grant number PI20/01052 and DTS22/00048).

Institutional Review Board Statement: The study was conducted in accordance with the Declaration of Helsinki and approved by the Ethics Committee for Clinical Research of Fundación Jiménez Díaz University Hospital (PIC 75/2016_FJD, 14/2/2017). The animal study protocol was approved by the Committee on Animal Ethics and Welfare of Research Institute-Fundación Jiménez Díaz University Hospital (PIC 63/2016_FJD, 31/5/2016).

Informed Consent Statement: Informed consent was obtained from all subjects involved in the study.

Data Availability Statement: The data that support the findings of this study are available from the corresponding author, P.V.-C., upon reasonable request.

Acknowledgments: The authors thank Oliver Shaw for revising the manuscript for aspects related to the English language and C. Robledo Montero for proteomics studies.

Conflicts of Interest: The authors declare no conflict of interest.

References

1. Buell-Gutbrod, R.; Gwin, K. Pathologic diagnosis, origin, and natural history of pseudomyxoma peritonei. *Am. Soc. Clin. Oncol. Educ. Book* **2013**, *33*, 221–225. [CrossRef] [PubMed]
2. Morera-Ocon, F.J.; Navarro-Campoy, C. History of pseudomyxoma peritonei from its origin to the first decades of the twenty-first century. *World J. Gastrointest. Surg.* **2019**, *11*, 358–364. [CrossRef] [PubMed]
3. Govaerts, K.; Lurvink, R.J.; De Hingh, I.H.J.T.; Van der Speeten, K.; Villeneuve, L.; Kusamura, S.; Kepenekian, V.; Deraco, M.; Glehen, O.; Moran, B.J.; et al. Appendiceal tumours and pseudomyxoma peritonei: Literature review with PSOGI/EURACAN clinical practice guidelines for diagnosis and treatment. *Eur. J. Surg. Oncol.* **2021**, *47*, 11–35. [CrossRef]

4. Arjona-Sánchez, Á.; Martínez-López, A.; Valenzuela-Molina, F.; Rufián-Andújar, B.; Rufián-Peña, S.; Casado-Adam, Á.; Sánchez-Hidalgo, J.M.; Rodríguez-Ortiz, L.; Medina-Fernández, F.J.; Díaz-López, C.; et al. A Proposal for Modification of the PSOGI Classification according to the Ki-67 Proliferation Index in Pseudomyxoma Peritonei. *Ann. Surg. Oncol.* **2022**, *29*, 126–136. [CrossRef]
5. Floriano, I.; Silvinato, A.; Reis, J.C.; Cafalli, C.; Bernardo, W.M. Efficacy and safety in the use of intraperitoneal hyperthermia chemotherapy and peritoneal cytoreductive surgery for pseudomyxoma peritonei from appendiceal neoplasm: A systematic review. *Clinics* **2022**, *77*, 100039. [CrossRef] [PubMed]
6. Lin, Y.L.; Li, Y. The Biological Synthesis and the Function of Mucin 2 in Pseudomyxoma Peritonei. *Cancer Manag. Res.* **2021**, *13*, 7909–7917. [CrossRef]
7. Pillai, K.; Akhter, J.; Mekkawy, A.; Chua, T.C.; Morris, D.L. Physical and chemical characteristics of mucin secreted by pseudomyxoma peritonei (PMP). *Int. J. Med. Sci.* **2017**, *14*, 18–28. [CrossRef]
8. Wen, H.K.; Valle, S.J.; Morris, D.L. Bromelain and acetylcysteine (BromAc®): A novel approach to the treatment of mucinous tumours. *Am. J. Cancer Res.* **2023**, *13*, 1522–1532.
9. Tong, M.; Jacobs, J.P.; McHardy, I.H.; Braun, J. Sampling of Intestinal Microbiota and Targeted Amplification of Bacterial 16S rRNA Genes for Microbial Ecologic Analysis. *Curr. Protoc. Immunol.* **2014**, *107*, 7–41. [CrossRef]
10. O'Connell, J.T.; Tomlinson, J.S.; Roberts, A.A.; McGonigle, K.F.; Barsky, S.H. Pseudomyxoma Peritonei Is a Disease of MUC2-Expressing Goblet Cells. *Am. J. Pathol.* **2002**, *161*, 551–564. [CrossRef]
11. Mohamed, F.; Gething, S.; Haiba, M.; Brun, E.A.; Sugarbaker, P.H. Clinically aggressive pseudomyxoma peritonei: A variant of a histologically indolent process. *J. Surg. Oncol.* **2004**, *86*, 10–15. [CrossRef] [PubMed]
12. Nonaka, D.; Kusamura, S.; Baratti, D.; Casali, P.; Younan, R.; Deraco, M. CDX-2 expression in pseudomyxoma peritonei: A clinicopathological study of 42 cases. *Histopathology* **2006**, *49*, 381–387. [CrossRef] [PubMed]
13. Baratti, D.; Kusamura, S.; Nonaka, D.; Cabras, A.D.; Laterza, B.; Deraco, M. Pseudomyxoma Peritonei. *Ann. Surg.* **2009**, *249*, 243–249. [CrossRef]
14. Mall, A.S.; Chirwa, N.; Govender, D.; Lotz, Z.; Tyler, M.; Rodrigues, J.; Kahn, D.; Goldberg, P. MUC2, MUC5AC and MUC5B in the mucus of a patient with pseudomyxoma peritonei: Biochemical and immunohistochemical study. *Pathol. Int.* **2007**, *57*, 537–547. [CrossRef]
15. Ferreira, C.R.; Carvalho, J.P.; Soares, F.A.; Siqueira, S.A.C.; Carvalho, F.M. Mucinous ovarian tumors associated with pseudomyxoma peritonei of adenomucinosis type: Immunohistochemical evidence that they are secondary tumors. *Int. J. Gynecol. Cancer* **2008**, *18*, 59–65. [CrossRef] [PubMed]
16. Guo, A.T.; Song, X.; Wei, L.X.; Zhao, P. Histological origin of pseudomyxoma peritonei in Chinese women: Clinicopathology and immunohistochemistry. *World J. Gastroenterol.* **2011**, *17*, 3531–3537. [CrossRef]
17. Chang, M.S.; Byeon, S.J.; Yoon, S.O.; Kim, B.H.; Lee, H.S.; Kang, G.H.; Kim, W.H.; Park, K.J. Leptin, MUC2 and mTOR in Appendiceal Mucinous Neoplasms. *Pathobiology* **2012**, *79*, 45–53. [CrossRef]
18. Breugelmans, T.; Oosterlinck, B.; Arras, W.; Ceuleers, H.; De Man, J.; Hold, G.L.; De Winter, B.Y.; Smet, A. The role of mucins in gastrointestinal barrier function during health and disease. *Lancet Gastroenterol. Hepatol.* **2022**, *7*, 455–471. [CrossRef]
19. Khamzina, Y.; King, M.C.; Nieroda, C.; Merrell, D.S.; Sardi, A.; Gushchin, V. The Role of Microorganisms in Appendiceal Pseudomyxoma Peritonei: A Review. *Curr. Oncol.* **2022**, *29*, 3576–3584. [CrossRef]
20. Arumugam, M.; Raes, J.; Pelletier, E.; Le Paslier, D.; Yamada, T.; Mende, D.R.; Fernandes, G.R.; Tap, J.; Bruls, T.; Batto, J.M.; et al. Enterotypes of the human gut microbiome. *Nature* **2011**, *473*, 174–180. [CrossRef]
21. Gilbreath, J.J.; Semino-Mora, C.; Friedline, C.J.; Liu, H.; Bodi, K.L.; McAvoy, T.J.; Francis, J.; Nieroda, C.; Sardi, A.; Dubois, A.; et al. A core microbiome associated with the peritoneal tumors of pseudomyxoma peritonei. *Orphanet J. Rare Dis.* **2013**, *8*, 105. [CrossRef]
22. Uhlén, M.; Fagerberg, L.; Hallström, B.M.; Lindskog, C.; Oksvold, P.; Mardinoglu, A.; Sivertsson, Å.; Kampf, C.; Sjöstedt, E.; Asplund, A.; et al. Tissue-based map of the human proteome. *Science* **2015**, *347*, 1260419. [CrossRef]
23. Dohrman, A.; Miyata, S.; Gallup, M.; Li, J.D.; Chapelin, C.; Coste, A.; Escudier, E.; Nadel, J.; Basbaum, C. Mucin gene (MUC 2 and MUC 5AC) upregulation by Gram-positive and Gram-negative bacteria. *Biochim. Biophys. Acta Mol. Basis Dis.* **1998**, *1406*, 251–259. [CrossRef] [PubMed]
24. Ben Mohamed, F.; Garcia-Verdugo, I.; Medina, M.; Balloy, V.; Chignard, M.; Ramphal, R.; Touqui, L. A Crucial Role of Flagellin in the Induction of Airway Mucus Production by *Pseudomonas aeruginosa*. *PLoS ONE* **2012**, *7*, e39888. [CrossRef]
25. García-Olmo, D.; Olmedillas-López, S.; Cortés-Guiral, D.; Villarejo, P.; López Rojo, I.; Guadalajara, H.; García Gómez-Heras, S.; García-Arranz, M. The role of mucin cell-free DNA detection as a new marker for the study of acellular pseudomyxoma peritonei of appendicular origin by liquid biopsy. *Ther. Adv. Med. Oncol.* **2020**, *12*, 175883592092823. [CrossRef] [PubMed]
26. Semino-Mora, C.; Testerman, T.L.; Liu, H.; Whitmire, J.M.; Studeman, K.; Jia, Y.; McAvoy, T.J.; Francis, J.; Nieroda, C.; Sardi, A.; et al. Antibiotic Treatment Decreases Microbial Burden Associated with Pseudomyxoma Peritonei and Affects β-Catenin Distribution. *Clin. Cancer Res.* **2013**, *19*, 3966–3976. [CrossRef]
27. Park, S.C.; Shimamura, I.; Fukunaga, M.; Mori, K.I.; Nakai, T. Isolation of Bacteriophages Specific to a Fish Pathogen, *Pseudomonas plecoglossicida*, as a Candidate for Disease Control. *Appl. Environ. Microbiol.* **2000**, *66*, 1416–1422. [CrossRef] [PubMed]
28. Nishimori, E.; Kita-Tsukamoto, K.; Wakabayashi, H. *Pseudomonas plecoglossicida* sp. nov., the causative agent of bacterial haemorrhagic ascites of ayu, *Plecoglossus altivelis*. *Int. J Syst. Evol. Microbiol.* **2000**, *50*, 83–89. [CrossRef]

29. Zhang, J.T.; Zhou, S.M.; An, S.W.; Chen, L.; Wang, G.L. Visceral granulomas in farmed large yellow croaker, *Larimichthys crocea* (Richardson), caused by a bacterial pathogen, *Pseudomonas plecoglossicida*. *J. Fish Dis.* **2014**, *37*, 113–121. [CrossRef]
30. Huang, L.; Zuo, Y.; Jiang, Q.; Su, Y.; Qin, Y.; Xu, X.; Zhao, L.; Yan, Q. A metabolomic investigation into the temperature-dependent virulence of *Pseudomonas plecoglossicida* from large yellow croaker (*Pseudosciaena crocea*). *J. Fish Dis.* **2019**, *42*, 431–446. [CrossRef]
31. Sun, Y.; Zhu, Z.; Weng, S.; He, J.; Dong, C. Characterization of a highly lethal barramundi (*Lates calcarifer*) model of *Pseudomonas plecoglossicida* infection. *Microb. Pathog.* **2020**, *149*, 104516. [CrossRef] [PubMed]
32. Li, C.H.; Xiong, J.B.; Ding, F.F.; Chen, J. Immune and gut bacterial successions of large yellow croaker (*Larimichthys crocea*) during *Pseudomonas plecoglossicida* infection. *Fish Shellfish Immunol.* **2020**, *99*, 176–183. [CrossRef] [PubMed]
33. Fernández, M.; Porcel, M.; de la Torre, J.; Molina-Henares, M.A.; Daddaoua, A.; Llamas, M.A.; Roca, A.; Carriel, V.; Garzón, I.; Ramos, J.L.; et al. Analysis of the pathogenic potential of nosocomial *Pseudomonas putida* strains. *Front. Microbiol.* **2015**, *6*, 871. [CrossRef] [PubMed]

Journal of
Clinical Medicine

MDPI

Article

Diagnostic Accuracy of Abdominal CT for Locally Advanced Colon Tumors: Can We Really Entrust Certain Decisions to the Reliability of CT?

Yaiza García del Álamo Hernández [1,†], Óscar Cano-Valderrama [2,†], Carlos Cerdán-Santacruz [1,*], Fernando Pereira Pérez [3], Inés Aldrey Cao [4], Sandra Núñez Fernández [4], Eduardo Álvarez Sarrado [5], Rosángela Obregón Reina [6], Paula Dujovne Lindenbaum [6], María Taboada Ameneiro [7], David Ambrona Zafra [8], Silvia Pérez Farré [8], Marta Pascual Damieta [9], Ricardo Frago Montanuy [10], Blas Flor Lorente [5], Sebastiano Biondo [10] and Collaborative Group for the Study of Metachronous Peritoneal Metastases of pT4 Colon Cancer [11,‡]

1 Colorectal Surgery Department, Hospital Universitario de la Princesa, Instituto de Investigación Sanitaria Princesa (IIS-IP), Universidad Autónoma de Madrid (UAM), 28006 Madrid, Spain
2 Colorectal Surgery Department, Complejo Hospitalario Universitario de Vigo, 36312 Vigo, Spain; oscarcanovalderrama@hotmail.com
3 General Surgery Department, Hospital de Fuenlabrada, 28942 Madrid, Spain; fernando.pereira@salud.madrid.org
4 Colorectal Surgery Department, Complexo Hospitalario Universitario de Ourense, 32005 Ourense, Spain; inesaldrey@hotmail.com (I.A.C.)
5 Colorectal Surgery Department, Hospital Politécnico Universitario la Fe, 46026 Valencia, Spain
6 Colorectal Surgery Department, Hospital General Universitario Gregorio Marañón, 28007 Madrid, Spain
7 Colorectal Surgery Department, Complejo Hospitalario Universitario de A Coruña (CHUAC), 15006 A Coruña, Spain; maria.taboada.ameneiro@sergas.es
8 Colorectal Surgery Department, Hospital Arnau de Vilanova de Lleida, 25198 Lleida, Spain
9 Colorectal Surgery Department, Hospital del Mar de Barcelona, 08003 Barcelona, Spain; mpascual@psmar.cat
10 Department of General and Digestive Surgery, Bellvitge University Hospital, University of Barcelona and IDIBELL, 08908 L'Hospitalet de Llobregat, Spain; sbn.biondo@gmail.com (S.B.)
11 Spanish Surgical Society Colorectal and Peritoneal Surgery Sections, 28006 Madrid, Spain
* Correspondence: carloscerdansantacruz@hotmail.com
† These authors contributed equally to this work.
‡ Collaborators of the Spanish PRS Collaborating Group are indicated in the Supplementary Materials section.

Abstract: Many different options of neoadjuvant treatments for advanced colon cancer are emerging. An accurate preoperative staging is crucial to select the most appropriate treatment option. A retrospective study was carried out on a national series of operated patients with T4 tumors. Considering the anatomo-pathological analysis of the surgical specimen as the gold standard, a diagnostic accuracy study was carried out on the variables T and N staging and the presence of peritoneal metastases (M1c). The parameters calculated were sensitivity, specificity, positive and negative predictive values, and positive and negative likelihood ratios, as well as the overall accuracy. A total of 50 centers participated in the study in which 1950 patients were analyzed. The sensitivity of CT for correct staging of T4 colon tumors was 57%. Regarding N staging, the overall accuracy was 63%, with a sensitivity of 64% and a specificity of 62%; however, the positive and negative likelihood ratios were 1.7 and 0.58, respectively. For the diagnosis of peritoneal metastases, the accuracy was 94.8%, with a sensitivity of 40% and specificity of 98%; in the case of peritoneal metastases, the positive and negative likelihood ratios were 24.4 and 0.61, respectively. The diagnostic accuracy of CT in the setting of advanced colon cancer still has some shortcomings for accurate diagnosis of stage T4, correct classification of lymph nodes, and preoperative detection of peritoneal metastases.

Keywords: advanced colon cancer; CT staging; diagnostic accuracy

1. Introduction

Up to 20–30% of colon cancer is diagnosed at locally advanced stages. Although the definition of this group of tumors is not unanimous, it generally comprises tumors classified as T3 with invasion of muscularis propria ≥ 5 mm, T4 with serosal involvement or direct invasion of adjacent structures, and tumors with regional nodal extension [1]. Certain patterns of peritoneal involvement have also been considered in this group of tumors due to similarities in prognosis [2]. Although it is obvious, it has to be taken into account that patients with peritoneal metastases is quite a wider group, and comparisons between both tumor groups should be performed with extreme caution. According to the National Comprehensive Cancer Network, 17% of diagnosed metastatic colon cancer patients present synchronous peritoneal metastases at diagnosis, of which 2% present metastases restricted to this location. Both locally advanced tumors and the presence of synchronous peritoneal metastases are associated with a worse prognosis with a negative impact on survival [3–5].

Due to the improvements in prognosis that are being achieved with some therapeutic strategies in certain clinical contexts, utilizing the correct staging is becoming increasingly important. Some examples of this may be the performance of extended D3 lymphadenectomy in certain colon cancers, especially on the right side, the possibility of administering neoadjuvant chemotherapy in locally advanced cases or even performing surgery with cytoreduction, and hyperthermic intraperitoneal chemotherapy in those cases of tumors with the presence of peritoneal metastases at diagnosis or with characteristics that confer a high risk of local or peritoneal recurrence, such as T4 tumors [6–11]. All these treatment options are not yet standard procedures, and therefore, studies are still needed to support their use, especially because they are aggressive treatments with a non-negligible morbi-mortality, which makes the proper selection of patients essential.

However, despite the evolution of therapeutics, the field of diagnostic evaluation in these cases has not undergone the same development. Several recent studies have shown that staging by abdominal CT can be misleading in a percentage of these locally advanced tumors, with a non-negligible risk of errors in preoperative staging, both over- and under-staging, with consequent errors in proper treatment planning [12,13]. The most challenging situations for reaching a correct diagnosis, i.e., some of the scenarios for which the selection of the most appropriate strategy is of utmost importance, can be considered to be the suspicion of a T4 tumor and the presence or absence of affected lymph nodes or peritoneal metastases [14–16]. Taking into account the existing difficulties for a correct diagnosis in reference institutions and in clinical studies, the aim of the present study was to analyze the diagnostic reliability of CT for locally advanced colon tumors in a routine clinical practice setting. This analysis could provide valuable information to better select candidate patients for certain aggressive therapeutic strategies in real-life contexts.

2. Materials and Methods

Local Clinical Research Ethics Committee (CREC) from Hospital de la Princesa (Madrid) approved this study (04/21-4398).

This study is a secondary analysis of an original study registered in ClinicalTrials.gov, number NCT05300789, in which the oncological outcome was investigated in a selected subgroup of pT4 colon cancer patients [17].

Patient consent was waived due to its retrospective and observational nature.

2.1. Design, Patients, and Variables

An observational retrospective multicenter trial was designed. A total of 50 different hospitals were enrolled in the project. This study was sponsored by the Spanish Surgical Society (Asociación Española de Cirujanos), both by the Colorectal and Peritoneal Surgery sections.

All consecutive patients operated on between 2015 and 2017 for colon cancer with curative intent, both elective and emergency operations, with pathological confirmation of pT4 stage adenocarcinoma, were included. Colon cancer was considered as the presence of tumors located in the large bowel at 15 cm above the anal verge. The exclusion criteria were as follows: patients younger than 18 years old, inability to achieve a whole tumor resection or palliative surgery (R2), patients without preoperative CT scan, pathological diagnosis of colon cancer other than adenocarcinoma (such as GIST, leiomyosarcomas, neuroendocrine tumors, or others), and patients with missing information.

Peritoneal metastases were defined a priori in the study protocol as follows: suspicion of any tumoral disease at the peritoneum, either single or multifocal, in the CT scan, and pathologically confirmed peritoneal metastasis as the gold standard for comparison.

Data were recorded by two senior staff members in each participant center. Demographic, preoperative, and operative data as well as pathological analysis based on 8th Edition of TNM classification [18] were recorded.

2.2. Evaluation of Radiological Studies

Exact details of the equipment, study protocols, and report were entirely at the discretion of the participating institutions based on best clinical practice [3]. In all but four hospitals, specific teams were appointed to evaluate abdominal radiological complementary tests, including CT scans, for the present study. Every determination acquired during planned CT scans for the staging of colon cancer patients was analyzed and informed within these specific units. Regarding determinations acquired during emergency situations, all of them were reported in this setting, but afterwards, in every institution, all the determinations were routinely re-evaluated by the abdominal imaging team in order to confirm or reinterpret the previously provided information.

2.3. Statistical Method

Qualitative variables are presented as numbers with their frequency distribution. Quantitative variables are represented as their mean and standard deviation (SD) or median and interquartile range (IQR) in case of asymmetry. The null hypothesis was rejected when the α or I error was <0.05. In order to assess the CT scan accuracy for the diagnosis of T4 colon malignancies, lymph node status, and peritoneal metastases, the calculated parameters were as follows: sensitivity (S), specificity (Sp), positive and negative predictive values (PPV and NPV, respectively), positive and negative likelihood ratios (PLR and NLR, respectively), and overall accuracy. All parameters are provided with a 95% confidence interval (CI).

The results are reported in accordance with the STARD (Standards for Reporting of Diagnostic Accuracy studies) Statement [19].

All calculations were performed using Stata 13.1 (StataCorp, College Station, TX, USA).

3. Results

3.1. Patients' Description and Radiological Findings

A total of 50 different hospitals participated in the study with a total sample record of 2546 patients with pT4 colon cancer. After the inclusion and exclusion criteria were applied, a final population of 1950 patients were analyzed (Figure 1).

Mean age was 70 years (SD 12 years), and 57% were male patients. Table 1 summarizes demographic, preoperative, and operative variables, and the most relevant postoperative outcomes. The most frequent initial clinical presentations from which colon cancer was diagnosed were obstructive symptoms in 484 cases (29.5%), followed by bleeding in 396 (24.2%), gastrointestinal transit disturbance in 207 (12.6%), and constitutional syndrome in 235 (14.3%).

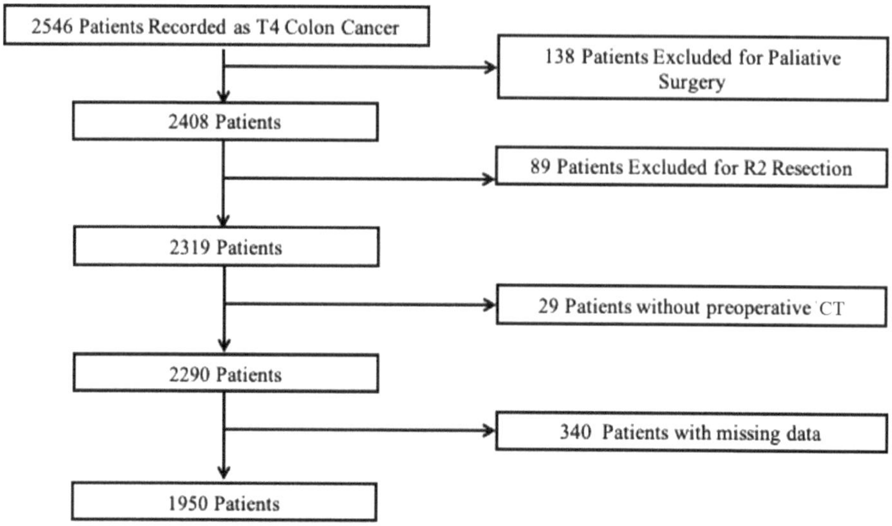

Figure 1. Flowchart detailing the selection of the patients in this study.

Table 1. Patients´ demographics and preoperative tumor characteristics.

		n	%
Age (Years) *		70.2	(SD 12.3)
Male		1115	57.2
ASA	I	85	4.4
	II	907	46.9
	III	846	43.8
	IV	95	4.9
BMI	<30	1217	77.2
	≥30	359	22.8
Asymptomatic		311	16
Symptomatology	Altered bowel transit	207	12.6
	Obstruction	484	29.5
	Constitutional syndrome	235	14.3
	Bleeding	396	24.2
	Others	317	19.3
Location	Right colon	851	43.6
	Left colon	1099	56.4
cT	T0–T1	85	4.4
	T2	114	5.8
	T3	641	32.9
	T4	1110	56.9
cN	N0	889	45.6
	N1	724	37.1
	N2	337	17.3
cM1		78	4

ASA: American Society of Anesthesiologist; BMI: body mass index. cT: clinical diagnosis for T stage. cN: clinical diagnosis for N stage. cM1: clinical diagnosis for M1 stage. * Data are expressed as mean and standard deviation.

All patients underwent preoperative abdominal CT. From the total number of patients, 1110 (56.9%) patients were classified to have T4 tumors, followed by 641 (32.9%) with T3,

114 (5.8%) with T2, and 85 (4.4%) with T0–T1 tumors. Nodal involvement was described in 1061 (54.4%) patients (37.1% N1 and 17.3% N2). Synchronous peritoneal metastases were diagnosed in 78 (4%) cases. Regarding tumor location, 1099 (56.4%) tumors were found in the left colon, with the remainder on the right side.

3.2. Operative Surgical Data and Pathological Assessment

The most common approach was laparotomy, performed in 1196 (61.3%) cases. The most frequent procedure was right hemicolectomy, performed in 802 (41.3%) patients, followed by sigmoidectomy in 581 (29.9%), and left hemicolectomy in 235 (12.1%). Emergency surgery was performed in 465 patients (23.9%) patients of the sample, among them obstruction was the most frequent cause (in 204 patients). A total of 605 (32.4%) patients required extended resection procedures during the intervention.

The histological variables are shown in Table 2. The predominant histological subtype was adenocarcinoma in 1728 tumors (88.6%). Most tumors were low grade (1545; 80.2%) and well (865; 45.5%) or moderately (680; 35.8%) differentiated. The margins were microscopically affected in 221 cases (11.3%). There were 261 (13.4%) cases with a finding of tumor perforation. Within the whole sample, 1487 (76.3%) tumors were T4a, while the remaining tumors were T4b. The mean number of lymph nodes retrieved in the surgical specimens was 21.5 (SD 12.8), with 1652 (84.8%) of the patients having 12 or more nodes evaluated. There were 1233 (63.2%) patients with positive adenopathy for malignancy. After the results of the anatomopathological study, 1396 (71.8%) patients received adjuvant chemotherapy.

Table 2. Operative data, pathological assessment, and adjuvant treatment details.

KERRYPNX		n	%
Type of surgery	Elective surgery	1485	76.2
	Emergency surgery	465	23.9
Surgical procedure	Right hemicolectomy	802	41.3
	Left hemicolectomy	235	12.1
	Sigmoidectomy	572	29.5
	Hartmann's surgery	136	7
	Others	195	10
Histological type	Adenocarcinoma	1728	88.6
	Signet ring cell/mucinous carcinoma	222	11.4
Differentiation grade	G1	865	45.5
	G2	680	35.8
	G3	357	18.8
Affected margins		221	11.3
Perineural invasion		708	36.9
Vascular invasion		822	42.8
Lymphatic invasion		876	45.8
Tumor perforation		261	13.4
T4a category		1487	76.3
N category	N0	717	36.8
	N1	700	35.9
	N2	533	27.3
M1c		120	6.1
Stage	II	626	32.3
	III	944	48.7
	IV	369	19
Adjuvant chemotherapy		1396	71.8

3.3. CT Scan Accuracy

The preoperative diagnosis established with abdominal CT on T and N staging (according to lymph node involvement) and the presence of synchronous peritoneal metastases (M1c), in relation to the final pathological diagnosis, is shown in Table 3. Data regarding CT diagnostic accuracy are shown in Table 4. The diagnostic sensitivity and the false negative rate (FNR) were calculated for the "T" staging of these pT4 tumors. The overall sensitivity was 56.9% (95% CI: 52.9–57.7%), while the sensitivity for the diagnosis of tumors categorized preoperatively as locally advanced (T3 and T4) was 89.8% (95% CI 88.5–91.1%).

Table 3. CT scan preoperative staging vs. histopathological assessment.

		Pathological Assessment		
		pT4		
CT Scan Diagnosis T category	cT1	85 (4)		
	cT2	114 (6)		
	cT3	641 (33)		
	cT4	1110 (57)		
	TOTAL	1950 (100)		
		Pathological Assessment		
		pN0	pN1/N2	
CT Scan Diagnosis N category	cN0	445	444	889
	cN1/N2	272	789	1061
	TOTAL	717	1233	1950
		Pathological Assessment		
		pM0	pM1c	
CT Scan Diagnosis M1c category	cM0	1800	72	1872
	cM1c	30	48	78
	TOTAL	1830	120	1950

The values obtained for the diagnostic ability of CT for pathologic lymph nodes (N+) were a sensitivity of 64% (95% CI 61.3–66.6%) and a specificity of 62.1% (95% CI 58.5–65.5%), with an overall accuracy of 63.3%. The positive likelihood ratio for the diagnosis of N+ was 1.7 (95% CI 1.5–1.9), while the negative likelihood ratio was 0.58 (95% CI 0.53–0.64).

For the diagnosis of peritoneal metastases, the sensitivity and specificity were 40% (95% CI 31.7–48.9%) and 98.4% (95% CI 97.7–98.8%), respectively, with an overall accuracy of 94.8%. The positive likelihood ratio for the diagnosis of synchronous peritoneal disease, M1c, was 24.4 (95% CI 17.68–30.5), while the negative likelihood ratio was 0.61 (95% CI 0.53–0.70).

The data about the CT scan accuracy, for stage T4, nodal stage, and peritoneal metastases, are summarized in Table 4.

Table 4. CT scan accuracy for pT4 tumors, N status, and M1c staging.

	T4 Category	
	Value (%)	95% CI
Sensitivity	57	55–59
FNR	43	41–45

Table 4. *Cont.*

	N Category	
	Value (%)	**95% CI**
Accuracy	63	61–65
Sensitivity	64.0	61.3–66.6
Specificity	62.1	58.5–65.5
PPV	74.4	71.7–76.9
NPV	50.1	46.8–53.3
PLR	1.7	1.5–1.9
NLR	0.58	0.53–0.64
	M1c Category	
	Value (%)	**95% CI**
Accuracy	94.8	93.7–95.7
Sensitivity	40	31.7–48.9
Specificity	98.4	97.7–98.8
PPV	61.5	50.4–71.6
NPV	96.2	95.2–96.9
PLR	24.4	16–37
NLR	0.61	0.53–0.70

95% CI: 95% confidence interval; FNR: false negative rate; PPV: positive predictive value; NPV: negative predictive value; PLR: positive likelihood ratio; NLR: negative likelihood ratio.

4. Discussion

In this study, based on a selected cohort of patients with pT4 colon tumors, the most advanced local stage possible, conventional abdominal CT has shown limited diagnostic accuracy, both in the characterization of the T4 stage and in the determination of affected lymph nodes (N+), and also in the diagnosis of synchronous peritoneal metastases.

In an era in which we are moving towards practically individualized medicine and in which patients are intended to be more and more involved in decisions about their treatment, obtaining the best diagnostic accuracy is a fundamental objective, especially because often there is no single standard treatment and the treatment offers and options are constantly increasing.

In the field of advanced colon cancer, certain strategies have flourished, aiming to administer preoperative oncological treatments that were classically administered post-operatively [11]. Although this approach is attractive, it should be noted that it may be associated with a significant risk of over-treatment. Some authors have estimated the risk of over-staging as 1 in every 12 diagnosed patients (95% CI, 9–16) [12]. This should be taken into consideration, not only because of the specific risks of these treatments and their toxicity, but also because of the potential oncological impact on the host, preoperatively altering the dynamics and biology of the tumor.

Although results are positive when locally advanced tumors in the broadest sense of their characterization (T3 tumors with >5 mm wall involvement and T4 tumors) are considered, the fine differentiation between the different T stages, the diagnostic reliability of the N category, and, above all, the possibility of an accurate diagnosis of the presence of synchronous peritoneal metastases as well as their preoperative characterization, are still unresolved diagnostic challenges.

The findings obtained in the present study have been previously reported by other studies that analyzed this topic, although with clinical designs different from the one chosen in our study [20,21].

Fernandez et al. [22] presented a retrospective study in 2019 that determined the diagnostic validity of abdominal CT for T and N staging of colon cancer. They included 150 patients who underwent right hemicolectomy with previous abdominal CT and were divided into two groups (early tumors vs. late tumors). They obtained diagnostic sensitivities of 50% for T1 and T2 tumors and 57% for T3 and T4 tumors. In the case of lymph node staging, the diagnostic parameters (sensitivity, specificity, PPV, and NPV) were 47%, 71%, 59%, and 61%, respectively. In both "N" and "T" staging, underdiagnosis was close to 50%; therefore, they concluded that only using this test for diagnosis could be insufficient. Olsen et al. [23] also retrospectively studied the diagnostic performance of CT, including 4832 colon cancer patients from a Danish national registry. The sensitivity for diagnosing T3-T4 tumors was 73%. The diagnostic parameters for N+ tumors were 57%, 66%, 50%, and 73% for sensitivity, specificity, PPV, and NPV, respectively. According to these results, they recommended caution when making therapeutic decisions based on conventional CT.

A meta-analysis published in 2016 by Nerad et al. [15] studied the sensitivity and specificity of CT for T and N staging; for T staging, they included 13 articles, obtaining 90% and 69%, respectively, while for N staging they included 16 articles, obtaining 71% and 67%, respectively. A differential analysis was carried out according to whether the thickness of the slices used in the CT was greater or less than 5 mm. This analysis provided better results in the second group. In our study, over-staging of tumors $\leq$ pT3 cannot be estimated as it only includes pT4 tumors. But in pT4 tumors and under real clinical practice conditions, preoperative CT underestimates the T4 category (classifying them as $\leq$T3) in 43% of cases. As for N, it classifies 36% of pN+ as N0 (false negative—FN). Conversely, 37.9% of pN0 were classified as N+ (false positive—FP). Therefore, both the risk of under-staging and over-staging are relevant for the N category.

Finally, we addressed in our study the diagnosis of synchronous peritoneal metastases. Our results, with a sensitivity of 40%, which means 60% of peritoneal metastases cases remain undiagnosed (FN), and a specificity of 98.4%, which means 1.6% of cases are mistakenly diagnosed to be positive for peritoneal metastases (FP), reflected the existing difficulty in the radiological diagnosis of peritoneal involvement. These figures are quite relevant, as under-estimation of peritoneal metastases might have devastating effects, while over-estimation might not. However, this aspect is the least studied in the literature, with most studies being heterogeneous (including studies of ovarian and other tumors of the upper gastrointestinal tract). Regarding colon cancer, there are few articles published including prospective samples from patients with peritoneal metastases found on abdominal CT who will undergo exploratory laparoscopy, so they calculate the diagnostic parameters with respect to the PCI (peritoneal cancer index). They have reported that CT scan underestimates the peritoneal extension of the disease, with the pelvis being the most underdiagnosed region [24–26].

In our opinion, it is quite noticeable that the likelihood ratio (LR) has not been used more extensively in the evaluation of CT as a diagnostic tool in this setting. Most common parameters, such as S, Sp, PPV, and NPV values, may not be good measures as they are influenced by the prevalence of the disease or the condition that is being rated in the population. On the contrary, the LR, which represents the ratio of the probability of a particular test result in patients with the disease and the probability of the same result in patients without the disease, is considered a powerful measure of the accuracy of diagnostic tests [25]. Consequently, the interpretation of the LR of a test reflects by how much the probability of presenting a disease increases or decreases depending on the result of a particular test. The closer to one the result of the LR calculations is, the lower is the impact of the diagnostic test employed on the post-test probability of the disease [25]. Based on these considerations, CT scan findings must be still considered with great caution in this context. On the one hand, the high PLR (more than 20) reflects a significant level of correct diagnosis of peritoneal metastases, although on the other hand, a low NLR (0.61) reflects a significant level of underdiagnosis of the disease under consideration. However, this is still more a potential intrinsic problem of the technology resolution and diagnostic capacity of the CT scan itself, more than that of the interpretation of the obtained images. The same problem was highlighted regarding N status based on this interpretation of likelihood ratios.

An accurate preoperative categorization of lymph nodes can be considered a cornerstone for the implementation of certain strategies and to take certain decisions, although it has been demonstrated once again that it is quite difficult to achieve, despite the constant efforts being taken for its improvement.

To alleviate the problems of diagnostic staging with conventional CT, other techniques have been proposed in recent years for the identification of locally advanced tumors, such as colonography, also known as virtual colonoscopy, PET-CT, and magnetic resonance imaging (MRI). Colonography is indicated in cases with poor endoscopic preparation or high anesthetic risk. According to some studies, this test has a sensitivity of diagnosing more than 80% of locally advanced T tumors. Some authors consider that the distension of the colon applied in this test, and its three-dimensional reconstruction, allow a better evaluation of the deep wall involvement [26]. The other proposed complementary test for the preoperative study of colon cancer is PET-CT. However, this test is not appropriate to determine the in-depth involvement of the intestinal wall since radionuclide uptake seems to be more related to tumor size than to infiltration. It should also be taken into account that its sensitivity and specificity for diagnosing lymph node involvement is close to 40% and 90%, respectively; therefore, its routine preoperative use is not recommended [27]. Finally, the use of MRI in diagnostic studies for the staging of rectal cancer has become routine in recent years. It has also been studied for colon cancer, and it has been found that this test can be more sensitive than conventional CT in discriminating early vs. locally advanced tumors [28,29]. Currently, the evidence is still insufficient to recommend MRI for the therapeutic planning of colon cancer, since the problem of correct lymph node staging is still present [30], and it is a more expensive test, which requires much more time for its performance, and the increase in its demand is difficult to sustain in clinical practice.

An outstanding issue to study the diagnostic performance of CT for locally advanced colon tumors is the absence of a formal definition of this subgroup of tumors according to the AJCC [31]. Many authors have considered T3 with extramural invasion of >5 mm and T4 as locally advanced tumors, in accordance with what has been used in studies on the effect of neoadjuvant chemotherapy for this tumor group [32,33]. Other studies, on the other hand, consider locally advanced tumors as those classified as T3 and T4, without differentiating the T3 group according to the depth of extramural involvement [21,34]. In the coming years, tools that use artificial intelligence and radiomics will probably be integrated with the current diagnostic means. Today, the use of these instruments is far from its adequate use in clinical practice, but these instruments have the potential to become diagnostic alternatives that may help solve the diagnostic problem in question in the future [35,36].

The study has some limitations such as the fact that it is a retrospective study, there is a lack of information regarding existing protocols for the acquisition and interpretation of the images, and the absence of a common radiological protocol or the lack of information regarding the necessity and accuracy of further diagnostic studies such as MRI or PET-CT in this context, and the aforementioned bias of including only tumors with a histological diagnosis of T4. Taking into account that colon cancer is quite a common condition, it is presumable that all the participating institutions in this study were aware of the best clinical practices and updated guidelines at the time of recording of the data. In addition, although guidelines exist, there is no unanimity in the interpretation of certain images or uniform diagnostic criteria in some circumstances, such as lymph node status or peritoneal metastasis. The present study, developed in a "real-life" setting, is a perfect reflection of the inconsistencies and weaknesses of this important issue, that is, preoperative advanced colon cancer staging. In spite of all this, the study's strengths are the large number of patients with locally advanced tumors included in this study and that these patients had not received any neoadjuvant treatment before inclusion in this study; therefore, their anatomopathological diagnosis was not altered due to previous therapies. Another novelty of the study is that it not only addresses T and N staging but also addresses the synchronous peritoneal involvement. Finally, we would also like to highlight the use of the likelihood ratio as a parameter of diagnostic utility of CT, as we consider that it is of great diagnostic value and has been scarcely used in the literature up to now.

5. Conclusions

The diagnostic accuracy of conventional CT as a preoperative assessment tool for locally advanced colon cancer is still limited for some aspects such as T staging, lymph nodes status, or the presence of synchronous peritoneal metastases. Research to improve preoperative staging should continue, and treatment decisions based on conventional CT should be taken cautiously in view of its risk–benefit analysis.

Supplementary Materials: The following supporting information can be downloaded at: https://www.mdpi.com/article/10.3390/jcm12216764/s1. Spanish collaboration group for the study of metachronous peritoneal metastases of pT4 colon cancer.

Author Contributions: Conceptualization, Y.G.d.Á.H., Ó.C.-V. and C.C.-S.; methodology, Ó.C.-V. and C.C.-S.; formal analysis, Ó.C.-V.; data curation, I.A.C., S.N.F., E.Á.S., R.O.R., P.D.L., M.T.A., D.A.Z., S.P.F., M.P.D., R.F.M. and Collaborative Group for the Study of Metachronous Peritoneal Metastases of pT4 Colon Cancer; writing—original draft preparation, Y.G.d.Á.H., Ó.C.-V. and C.C.-S.; writing—review and editing, F.P.P., B.F.L. and S.B. All authors have read and agreed to the published version of the manuscript.

Funding: This research received no external funding.

Institutional Review Board Statement: The study was conducted in accordance with the Declaration of Helsinki and approved by the Local Clinical Research Ethics Committee (CREC) of Hospital de la Princesa in Madrid (Protocol ID number: 04/21-4398).

Informed Consent Statement: Patient consent was waived due to its retrospective and observational nature.

Data Availability Statement: All data and materials have been made publicly available through the Mendeley Data repository and can be accessed at Cerdán Santacruz, Carlos (2022), "Metachronous peritoneal carcinomatosis after pT4 colon cancer patients", Mendeley Data, V2, doi: 10.17632/k28wpghcts.2.

Acknowledgments: We also thank Manolo Gómez Gutiérrez from Instituto de Investigación Sanitaria Princesa (IIS-IP) for the professional English editing of the manuscript.

Conflicts of Interest: The authors declare no conflict of interest.

References

1. Gosavi, R.; Chia, C.; Michael, M.; Heriot, A.G.; Warrier, S.K.; Kong, J.C. Neoadjuvant chemotherapy in locally advanced colon cancer: A systematic review and meta-analysis. *Int. J. Color. Dis.* **2021**, *36*, 2063–2070. [CrossRef] [PubMed]
2. Hameed, S.A.; Kusters, I.S.; Khan, M.; Matz, M. Colon cancer survival in California from 2004 to 2011 by stage at diagnosis, sex, race/ethnicity, and socioeconomic status. *Cancer Epidemiol.* **2021**, *72*, 101901. [CrossRef] [PubMed]
3. Benson, A.B.; Venook, A.P.; Al-Hawary, M.M.; Arain, M.A.; Chen, Y.J.; Ciombor, K.K.; Cohen, S.; Cooper, H.S.; Deming, D.; Farkas, L.; et al. Colon Cancer, Version 2.2021, NCCN Clinical Practice Guidelines in Oncology. *J. Natl. Compr. Cancer Netw.* **2021**, *19*, 329–359. [CrossRef] [PubMed]
4. Brouwer, N.P.; Van der Kruijssen, D.E.; Hugen, N.; de Hingh, I.H.; Nagtegaal, I.D.; Verhoeven, R.H.; Koopman, M.; de Wilt, J.H. The Impact of Primary Tumor Location in Synchronous Metastatic Colorectal Cancer: Differences in Metastatic Sites and Survival. *Ann. Surg. Oncol.* **2020**, *27*, 1580–1588. [CrossRef]
5. Grothey, A.; Sobrero, A.F.; Shields, A.F.; Yoshino, T.; Paul, J.; Taieb, J.; Souglakos, J.; Shi, Q.; Kerr, R.; Labianca, R.; et al. Duration of Adjuvant Chemotherapy for Stage III Colon Cancer. *N. Engl. J. Med.* **2018**, *378*, 1177–1188. [CrossRef] [PubMed]
6. Arjona-Sánchez, A.; Espinosa-Redondo, E.; Gutiérrez-Calvo, A.; Segura-Sampedro, J.J.; Pérez-Viejo, E.; Concepción-Martín, V.; Sánchez-García, S.; García-Fadrique, A.; Prieto-Nieto, I.; Barrios-Sanchez, P.; et al. Efficacy and Safety of Intraoperative Hyperthermic Intraperitoneal Chemotherapy for Locally Advanced Colon Cancer: A Phase 3 Randomized Clinical Trial. *JAMA Surg.* **2023**, *158*, 683–691. [CrossRef] [PubMed]
7. Cheong, C.K.; Nistala, K.R.Y.; Ng, C.H.; Syn, N.; Chang, H.S.Y.; Sundar, R.; Yang, S.Y.; Chong, C.S. Neoadjuvant therapy in locally advanced colon cancer: A meta-analysis and systematic review. *J. Gastrointest. Oncol.* **2020**, *11*, 847–857. [CrossRef] [PubMed]

8. Eng, O.S.; Turaga, K.K. Cytoreduction and hyperthermic intraperitoneal chemotherapy in metastatic colorectal cancer. *J. Surg. Oncol.* **2019**, *119*, 613–615. [CrossRef]
9. Konishi, T.; You, Y.N. Complete Mesocolic Excision and Extent of Lymphadenectomy for the Treatment of Colon Cancer. *Surg. Oncol. Clin. N. Am.* **2022**, *31*, 293–306. [CrossRef]
10. Quénet, F.; Elias, D.; Roca, L.; Goéré, D.; Ghouti, L.; Pocard, M.; Facy, O.; Arvieux, C.; Lorimier, G.; Pezet, D.; et al. Cytoreductive surgery plus hyperthermic intraperitoneal chemotherapy versus cytoreductive surgery alone for colorectal peritoneal metastases (PRODIGE 7): A multicentre, randomised, open-label, phase 3 trial. *Lancet Oncol.* **2021**, *22*, 256–266. [CrossRef]
11. Morton, D.; Seymour, M.; Magill, L.; Handley, K.; Glasbey, J.; Glimelius, B.; Palmer, A.; Seligmann, J.; Laurberg, S.; Murakami, K.; et al. Preoperative Chemotherapy for Operable Colon Cancer: Mature Results of an International Randomized Controlled Trial. *J. Clin. Oncol.* **2023**, *41*, 1541–1552. [CrossRef]
12. Elibol, F.D.; Obuz, F.; Sokmen, S.; Terzi, C.; Canda, A.E.; Sagol, O.; Sarioglu, S. The role of multidetector CT in local staging and evaluation of retroperitoneal surgical margin involvement in colon cancer. *Diagn. Interv. Radiol.* **2016**, *22*, 5–12. [CrossRef] [PubMed]
13. Malmstrøm, M.L.; Brisling, S.; Klausen, T.W.; Săftoiu, A.; Perner, T.; Vilmann, P.; Gögenur, I. Staging with computed tomography of patients with colon cancer. *Int. J. Color. Dis.* **2018**, *33*, 9–17. [CrossRef] [PubMed]
14. Leufkens, A.M.; van den Bosch, M.A.; van Leeuwen, M.S.; Siersema, P.D. Diagnostic accuracy of computed tomography for colon cancer staging: A systematic review. *Scand. J. Gastroenterol.* **2011**, *46*, 887–894. [CrossRef] [PubMed]
15. Nerad, E.; Lahaye, M.J.; Maas, M.; Nelemans, P.; Bakers, F.C.H.; Beets, G.L.; Beets-Tan, R.G.H. Diagnostic Accuracy of CT for Local Staging of Colon Cancer: A Systematic Review and Meta-Analysis. *AJR Am. J. Roentgenol.* **2016**, *207*, 984–995. [CrossRef] [PubMed]
16. Panagiotopoulou, P.B.; Courcoutsakis, N.; Tentes, A.; Prassopoulos, P. CT imaging of peritoneal carcinomatosis with surgical correlation: A pictorial review. *Insights Imaging* **2021**, *12*, 168. [CrossRef] [PubMed]
17. Cerdán-Santacruz, C.; Cano-Valderrama, Ó.; del Moral, S.; Pérez, F.P.; Lorente, B.F.; Biondo, S.; Caro, C.R.; Marchán, S.J.d.L.G.; López, F.F.; Novo, M.P.; et al. Epidemiology, oncologic results and risk stratification model for metachronous peritoneal metastases after surgery for pT4 colon cancers: Results from an observational retrospective multicentre long-term follow-up study. *Tech. Coloproctol.* **2023**, *27*, 1025–1036. [CrossRef] [PubMed]
18. Byrd, D.R.; Brookland, R.K.; Washington, M.K.; Gershenwald, J.E.; Compton, C.C.; Hess, K.R.; Sullivan, D.C.; Jessup, J.M. *AJCC Cancer Staging Manual*; Springer: New York, NY, USA, 2017; Volume 20, pp. 251–274.
19. Bossuyt, P.M.; Reitsma, J.B.; Bruns, D.E.; Gatsonis, C.A.; Glasziou, P.P.; Irwig, L.; Lijmer, J.G.; Moher, D.; Rennie, D.; de Vet, H.C.; et al. STARD 2015: An Updated List of Essential Items for Reporting Diagnostic Accuracy Studies. *Radiology.* **2015**, *277*, 826–832. [CrossRef] [PubMed]
20. Norgaard, A.; Dam, C.; Jakobsen, A.; Ploen, J.; Lindebjerg, J.; Rafaelsen, S.R. Selection of colon cancer patients for neoadjuvant chemotherapy by preoperative CT scan. *Scand. J. Gastroenterol.* **2014**, *49*, 202–208. [CrossRef]
21. Wiegering, A.; Kunz, M.; Hussein, M.; Klein, I.; Wiegering, V.; Uthe, F.W.; Dietz, U.A.; Jurowich, C.; Bley, T.; Dandekar, T.; et al. Diagnostic value of preoperative CT scan to stratify colon cancer for neoadjuvant therapy. *Int. J. Color. Dis.* **2015**, *30*, 1067–1073. [CrossRef]
22. Fernandez, L.M.; Parlade, A.J.; Wasser, E.J.; Dasilva, G.; de Azevedo, R.U.; Ortega, C.D.; Perez, R.O.; Habr-Gama, A.; Berho, M.; Wexner, S.D. How Reliable Is CT Scan in Staging Right Colon Cancer? *Dis. Colon. Rectum.* **2019**, *62*, 960–964. [CrossRef] [PubMed]
23. Olsen, A.S.F.; Gundestrup, A.K.; Kleif, J.; Thanon, T.; Bertelsen, C.A. Accuracy of preoperative staging with multidetector computed tomography in colon cancer. *Color. Dis.* **2021**, *23*, 680–688. [CrossRef] [PubMed]
24. Esquivel, J.; Chua, T.; Stojadinovic, A.; Melero, J.T.; Levine, E.; Gutman, M.; Howard, R.; Piso, P.; Nissan, A.; Gomez-Portilla, A.; et al. Accuracy and clinical relevance of computed tomography scan interpretation of peritoneal cancer index in colorectal cancer peritoneal carcinomatosis: A multi-institutional study. *J. Surg. Oncol.* **2010**, *102*, 565–570. [CrossRef] [PubMed]
25. Hayden, S.R.; Brown, M.D. Likelihood ratio: A powerful tool for incorporating the results of a diagnostic test into clinical decisionmaking. *Ann. Emerg. Med.* **1999**, *33*, 575–580. [CrossRef] [PubMed]
26. Maupoey Ibanez, J.; Pamies Guilabert, J.; Frasson, M.; Bosca Robledo, A.; Giner Segura, F.; Garcia-Granero Ximenez, E. Accuracy of CT colonography in the preoperative staging of colon cancer: A prospective study of 217 patients. *Color. Dis.* **2019**, *21*, 1151–1163. [CrossRef] [PubMed]
27. Kijima, S.; Sasaki, T.; Nagata, K.; Utano, K.; Lefor, A.T.; Sugimoto, H. Preoperative evaluation of colorectal cancer using CT colonography, MRI, and PET/CT. *World J. Gastroenterol.* **2014**, *20*, 16964–16975. [CrossRef] [PubMed]
28. Liu, L.H.; Lv, H.; Wang, Z.C.; Rao, S.X.; Zeng, M.S. Performance comparison between MRI and CT for local staging of sigmoid and descending colon cancer. *Eur. J. Radiol.* **2019**, *121*, 108741. [CrossRef]
29. Rafaelsen, S.R.; Dam, C.; Vagn-Hansen, C.; Møller, J.; Rahr, H.B.; Sjöström, M.; Lindebjerg, J.; Hansen, T.F.; Pedersen, M.R.V. CT and 3 Tesla MRI in the TN Staging of Colon Cancer: A Prospective, Blind Study. *Curr. Oncol.* **2022**, *29*, 1069–1079. [CrossRef]
30. Stelzner, S.; Ruppert, R.; Kube, R.; Strassburg, J.; Lewin, A.; Baral, J.; Maurer, C.A.; Sauer, J.; Lauscher, J.; Winde, G.; et al. Selection of patients with rectal cancer for neoadjuvant therapy using pre-therapeutic MRI—Results from OCUM trial. *Eur. J. Radiol.* **2022**, *147*, 110113. [CrossRef]
31. Weiser, M.R. AJCC 8th Edition: Colorectal Cancer. *Ann. Surg. Oncol.* **2018**, *25*, 1454–1455. [CrossRef]

32. Davey, M.G.; Amir, A.H.; Ryan, O.K.; Donnelly, M.; Donlon, N.E.; Regan, M.; Meshkat, B.; Nugent, E.; Joyce, M.; Hogan, A.M. Evaluating the oncological safety of neoadjuvant chemotherapy in locally advanced colon carcinoma: A systematic review and meta-analysis of randomised clinical trials and propensity-matched studies. *Int. J. Color. Dis.* **2023**, *38*, 193. [CrossRef]
33. Jakobsen, A.; Andersen, F.; Fischer, A.; Jensen, L.H.; Jørgensen, J.C.R.; Larsen, O.; Lindebjerg, J.; Pløen, J.; Rafaelsen, S.R.; Vilandt, J. Neoadjuvant chemotherapy in locally advanced colon cancer. A phase II trial. *Acta Oncol.* **2015**, *54*, 1747–1753. [CrossRef]
34. Silva, R.; Hamidi, M.; Omesiete, P.; Osman, F.; Charlton, C.; Banerjee, S.; Estrada, T.; Nfonsam, V. Does preoperative neoadjuvant chemotherapy impact short-term surgical outcomes in patients with locally advanced colon cancer? *Int. J. Color. Dis.* **2021**, *36*, 2127–2134. [CrossRef]
35. Dominguez-Prieto, V.; Barambio-Buendia, J.; Vizarreta-Figueroa, A.T.; Meliga, C.; Guijo-Castellano, I.; Villarejo-Campos, P. Value of three-dimensional reconstruction for non-invasive estimation of PCI in patients with peritoneal carcinomatosis of colorectal origin: A proof of concept. *Cir. Esp. (Engl. Ed.)* **2023**, *in press*. [CrossRef]
36. Garcia-Granero, A.; Mc-Farlane, S.J.; Cuesta, M.G.; Gonzalez-Argente, F.X. Application of 3D-reconstruction and artificial intelligence for complete mesocolic excision and D3 lymphadenectomy in colon cancer. *Cir. Esp. (Engl. Ed.)* **2023**, *101*, 359–368. [CrossRef] [PubMed]

Journal of
Clinical Medicine

MDPI

Article

Follow-up for More than 10 Years of Patients with Peritoneal Metastases Treated with Cytoreductive Surgery + Hyperthermic Intraperitoneal Chemotherapy in a Specialized Unit

Alba Fernández-Candela [1], Pedro Bretcha-Boix [1,*], Juan Carlos Ruíz Ramírez [2], Alejandro Paz [1], Paula Munoz [1], Miguel A. Ortega [3,4], Melchor Álvarez-Mon [4] and José Farré-Alegre [1]

1 Peritoneal Carcinomatosis Unit, General Surgery Department, Hospital Quironsalud Torrevieja, 03184 Torrevieja, Spain; alba.fernandezca@quironsalud.es (A.F.-C.); alejandro.paz@quironsalud.es (A.P.); paula.munozm@quironsalud.es (P.M.); jose.farre@quironsalud.es (J.F.-A.)
2 Pharmacy Department, Hospital Quironsalud Torrevieja, 03184 Torrevieja, Spain; juan.ruizram@quironsalud.es
3 Department of Medicine and Medical Specialties, Faculty of Medicine and Health Sciences, University of Alcalá, 28801 Alcalá de Henares, Spain; miguel.angel.ortega92@gmail.com
4 Ramón y Cajal Institute of Sanitary Research, 28034 Madrid, Spain; mademons@gmail.com
* Correspondence: pedro.bretcha@quironsalud.es

Abstract: Cytoreductive surgery (CRS) and hyperthermic intraperitoneal chemotherapy (HIPEC) have demonstrated their impact on disease-free survival (DFS) and overall survival (OS) of patients with peritoneal metastases (PM). However, prior literature lacks evidence regarding any follow-up beyond 5 years. In this study, we analyse long-term OS and DFS (more than 10 years of follow-up) of patients undergoing CRS + HIPEC in a specialized unit. We conducted a retrospective study that included only patients who underwent CRS + HIPEC from January 2001 to May 2012. Data collection was conducted by reviewing medical records and telephone calls to patients or relatives. A total of 86 patients were included. The mean PCI was nine (range 0–39) and complete cytoreduction (CC-0) was reached in 80% of patients. Postoperative complications Clavien–Dindo III-IV occurred in 27.9% of patients and the 30-day mortality rate was 2.3%. After 10 years of actual follow-up, OS was 33.7% and DFS was 31.4%. Considering the historical context in which the standard of care for patients with PM was palliation, the results obtained show that CRS + HIPEC was a valid option, with morbimortality comparable to other major abdominal surgeries and encouraging survival results, since, after 10 years of follow-up, almost one-third of patients are still alive and disease-free.

Keywords: peritoneal metastases; long-term follow-up; overall survival; free-disease survival; cytorreductive surgery; hyperthermic intraperitoneal chemotherapy; peritoneal carcinomatosis

1. Introduction

During the last two decades, cytoreductive surgery (CRS) and hyperthermic intraperitoneal chemotherapy (HIPEC) have changed the prognosis of patients with peritoneal metastases (PM). Patients with this condition were considered terminal and showed a median survival rate between 3 and 9 months depending on the primary tumour involved [1–4]. Nevertheless, in 2003, Verwaal et al. [5] published a randomized trial in which patients with colorectal PM undergoing CRS plus HIPEC showed a median survival rate of 22.6 months versus 12.6 months in patients following standard systemic chemotherapy ($p = 0.032$). These findings were confirmed by Glehen et al. [6] in 2004, who also concluded that complete cytoreductive surgery was the most important prognostic indicator. Similar results were published regarding ovarian cancer [7], gastric cancer [8], small bowel mucinous adenocarcinoma [9] and pseudomyxoma peritonei [10].

Following this favourable data, many institutions implemented this technique around the world, including Spain. Our health center, was one of the nine Spanish centers that started a specialized unit in 2001 [11]. Currently, after 20 years of experience, some centers have published their results [12,13], including all patients that have undergone CRS until now, with a heterogeneous follow-up period ranging from 1 year to 20 years. Only Kim et al. [14] have published results including a homogeneous follow-up period with 88.3% of patients with ten or more years of follow-up. According to that study, only ovarian PM patients were included and they obtained a ten-year survival rate of 19.3% in the CRS group versus 9.1% in the neoadjuvant chemotherapy group ($p < 0.001$).

The aim of our study is to analyse overall survival and disease-free survival rates after 10 or more years of follow-up in patients with PM that underwent CRS and HIPEC in our specialized unit.

2. Materials and Methods

2.1. Study Population

All patients treated for peritoneal metastases within a peritoneal surface malignancies program at the Quironsalud Torrevieja Hospital from January 2001 to May 2012 were initially considered. Finally, only those who met the selection criteria and had a complete follow-up were included. A retrospective cohort study was conducted from a prospectively gathered database. In May 2022 all patients included were contacted by phone to establish their health status.

2.2. Selection Criteria

Patients with acceptable performance status (ECOG < 2), age between 18–70 years old, live expectancy > 12 weeks, adequate haematological count (PNN $\geq 1.5 \times 10^9$, platelets $\geq 100 \times 10^9/L$) and correct hepatic function (total bilirubin ≤ 1.5, AST (GOT) and ALT (GPT) ≤ 3, alkaline phosphatase ≤ 3) and absence of retroperitoneal lymph node disease, extraperitoneal metastases, intestinal occlusion and serious heart/lung/liver/kidney disease, were included in the study.

Patients with mesenteric retraction in CT images, bladder infiltration, extra abdominal metastasis or unresectable liver metastases, another malignant tumour, multiple intestinal obstructions or active infection, were excluded.

2.3. Patient Data

Demographic variables were obtained, including age, sex, carcinomatosis origin and neoadjuvant chemotherapy. Neoadjuvant therapy was guided by tumour origin, therefore, colorectal patients followed the FOLFOX scheme (folinic acid + 5-florouracil + oxaliplatin), gastric patients followed the FLOT scheme (5-florouracil + leucovorin + oxaliplatin + docetaxel) and ovarian patients received carboplatin + taxol. Surgical variables such as peritoneal cancer index (PCI), grade of cytoreduction (CCS) and number of reinterventions, were also gathered. The PCI was categorized as low (1–9), medium (10–19) and high ($\geq$20). Clavien–Dindo classification [15] was followed to grade the 30-day and in-hospital postoperative complications and were subclassified as none (I), minor (II) and major (III–V). Hospital length of stay was also included.

2.4. Procedure

After monitoring the patient and administering a balanced general anaesthetic, a medial xipho-pubic laparotomy was performed to carefully examine the abdominal cavity. This allowed us to obtain the tumour load as well as the PCI, following Sugarbaker's method in which the abdomen is divided into 13 areas (0–12). We took biopsies from every area and cytological samples. The resection of the primary tumour was completed according to oncological criteria (R0 margins and lymphadenectomy), as well as peritonectomies and debulking when carcinomatosis was present, if not, we did not perform extensive systematic peritonectomies. Regarding mesenteric peritoneum metastases, we conducted acceptable small bowel resections in areas of maximum tumour volume and small implants were fulgurated with electrocautery. If no macroscopic implants were left, the cytoreduction was considered complete (CC-0). If residual implants remained, the cytoreduction was considered CC-1 when they were <2.5 mm, CC-2 when they were between 2.5 mm and 2.5 cm, and CC-3 when they were >2.5 cm [16]. The anastomoses were performed after the HIPEC was applied using Sugarbaker's open coliseum technique. We connected four 36-Fr drains to a continuous closed circuit and placed two intraperitoneal thermal probes to obtain an accurate temperature feedback. An extracorporeal circulation machine (Performer Rand®, Modena, Italy) delivered the perfusate at a flow of 500 mL/min and the heat exchanger raised the temperature of the fluid to 48 °C. Once we obtained this temperature, we initiated the drug administration, diluted in 3–5 L of 5% dextrose peritoneal dialysis fluid. The choice of drug depended on the primary tumour, as well as the length of the perfusion. In colorectal and appendicular tumours, we followed Sugarbaker's protocol and administered 12.5 mg/m^2 in women and 15 mg/m^2 in men of mitomycin C for 90 min; after Elias et al. [17] study, we changed protocol to 460 mg/m^2 of intraperitoneal oxaliplatin during 30 min, with an intravenous bolus of 600 mg of 5-fluoracil 30 min prior to infusion. Originally, for ovarian tumours we would administer Taxol for 60 min, but after Elias et al., we changed the protocol to oxaliplatin or cisplatin + doxorubicin or Taxol for 90 min. In gastric tumours and mesothelioma, we employed oxaliplatin for 30 min. The surgeon distributed the fluid in the cavity periodically during perfusion, and the hemodynamic response of the patient was carefully monitored. The liquid temperature in the abdominal cavity fluctuated between 42° and 43 °C. Subsequently, the liquid was drained and a peritoneal lavage was performed. Twenty-four hours later, early postoperative intraperitoneal chemotherapy (EPIC) was initiated with 650 mg/m^2 of 5-FU. The dose was kept for 23 h in the peritoneum and administered daily for 5 consecutive days. EPIC was administered until 2008 to all patients as a standard of care during this period.

2.5. Follow-up

All patients were seen at the outpatient clinic by oncologists and surgeons every 3 months for the first 2 years, every 6 months until 5 years after the surgery, and once a year thereafter. The follow-up consisted of physical examination and measurement of serum tumour markers on every visit and thoracoabdominal CT scans on alternative visits.

Follow-up after 10 years from the surgery was carried out by reviewing medical records and by phone. Patients were classified as alive and disease-free, alive but with disease, dead due to the disease (PM) or dead due to other causes. The date of relapse and date of death were also gathered. A follow-up was considered complete either through a successful contact by phone with the patient or relatives or knowledge of the date of death of the patient.

2.6. Statistical Analysis

The Competing Risk Analysis was used to calculate cumulative incidence of death (CID) and cumulative incidence of recurrence (CIR). CID encompassed from the date of the first CRS + HIPEC until the patient's death by cancer or until the last follow-up. CIR included from the date of CRS + HIPEC until the first patient's recurrence or until the last follow-up. Continuous variables were expressed as mean values (range). Categorical data were given as frequencies and proportions. All statistical analyses were conducted by IBM SPSS Statistics (version 27) and R version 4.3.0 (R Core Team, 2023) using package cmprsk (version 2.2-11—Gray B, 2021) for analysis of competing risk.

3. Results

3.1. Study Population and Surgical Outcomes

During the period between January 2001 and May 2012, many patients were evaluated in our specialized unit, but only 88 met the selection criteria for CRS + HIPEC. Finally, the complete follow-up was achieved in 86 patients, who are included in our sample. Of those 86 patients, twenty-three were men (26.7%) and sixty-three women (73.3%), with an overall mean age of 56 years old. Baseline and surgical characteristics are described in Table 1.

Table 1. Baseline and surgical characteristics.

	n = 86
Age	56 (24–78)
Sex	
Men	23 (26.7%)
Women	63 (73.3%)
Neoadjuvant therapy	
No	12 (14%)
Yes	74 (86%)
Origin	
Ovarian	38 (44.2%)
Colorectal	31 (36%)
Gastric	9 (10.5%)
Appendicular	5 (5.8%)
Mesothelioma	3 (3.5%)
PCI (mean)	9 (0–39)
PCI	
0	22 (26.2%)
1–9	33 (39.3%)
10–19	15 (17.9%)
≥20	14 (16.7%)
PCI 0	
Ovarian	10 (45%)
Colorectal	7 (31.81%)
Gastric	4 (18.18%)
Mesothelioma	1 (4.55%)
Cytoreduction	
Complete (CC-0)	68 (80%)
Optimal (CC-1)	9 (10.6%)
Incomplete (CC-2)	7 (8.2%)
Non-resectable (CC-3)	1 (1.2%)
Type of surgery	
Primary tumor	61 (70.9%)
Persistence	2 (2.3%)
Recurrence	15 (17.4%)
Second look	8 (9.3%)
HIPEC	
Oxaliplatin	55 (64.7%)
Mytomicin C	14 (16.5%)
Taxol	11 (12.9%)
Carboplatin	2 (2.4%)
Carboplatin + taxol	1 (1.2%)
Cisplatin + Doxorubicin	1 (1.2%)
Oxaliplatin + Doxorubicin	1 (1.2%)
EPIC	
No	14 (16.3%)
Yes	72 (83.7%)

Data are presented as mean (range) for continuous measures; number (%) for categorical measures. PCI: Peritoneal cancer index; HIPEC: hyperthermic intraperitoneal chemotherapy; EPIC: early postoperative intraperitoneal chemotherapy.

Ovarian cancer was the most common peritoneal metastase origin (44.2%), followed by colorectal cancer (36%) and gastric cancer (10.5%). Mean PCI was 9, ranging from 0 to 39, and complete cytoreduction (CC-0) was achieved in 80% of patients. As far as intraperitoneal chemotherapy drugs are concerned, oxaliplatin was the most used (64.7%), followed by mitomycin C (16.5%) and Taxol (12.9%).

3.2. Postoperative Outcomes

Postoperative complications occurred in 53.5% of patients, with 27.9% of major complications (Clavien–Dindo III–VI). The 30-day mortality rate was 2.3% and the mean postoperative hospital stay was 17 days. Details are outlined in Table 2.

Table 2. Postoperative outcomes.

	n = 86
Clavien–Dindo classification	
Grade I	40 (46.5%)
Grade II	20 (23.3%)
Grade IIIa	7 (8.1%)
Grade IIIb	9 (10.5%)
Grade IVa	6 (7%)
Grade IVb	2 (2.3%)
Grade V	2 (2.3%)
Clavien–Dindo categories	
No morbidity	40 (46.5%)
Minor morbidity	20 (23.3%)
Major morbidity	26 (27.9%)
In hospital stay	17 (4–63)
30-day mortality	2.3%
Reintervention	
No	72 (83.7%)
Yes	13 (15.1%)

Data are presented as number (%) for categorical measures and mean (range) for continuous measures.

3.3. Survival Outcomes

The median follow-up period was 66 months. The disease-free survival (DFS) curve is shown in Figure 1. The overall median DFS was 19 months with a 12- and 36- months DFS of 62.8% and 34.6%, respectively.

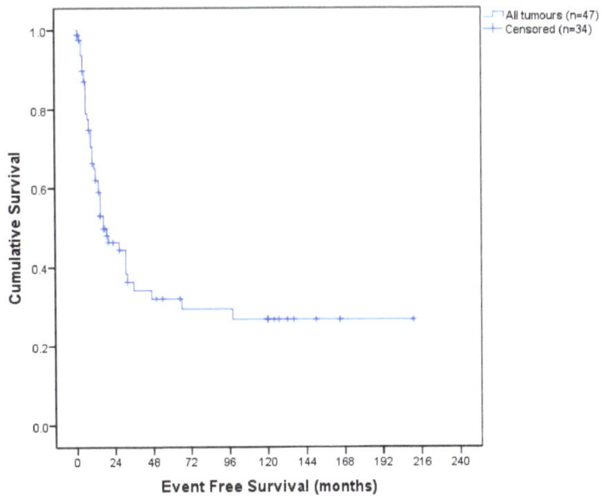

Figure 1. Disease-free survival curve.

The overall survival (OS) curve is shown in Figure 2. The median OS was 29 months, with a 12- and 36-month OS of 81.8% and 47.7%, respectively. After a 10-year follow-up, OS was 33.7% and DFS was 31.4%. At the time we conducted the survey (May 2022), 27 patients were alive and disease-free.

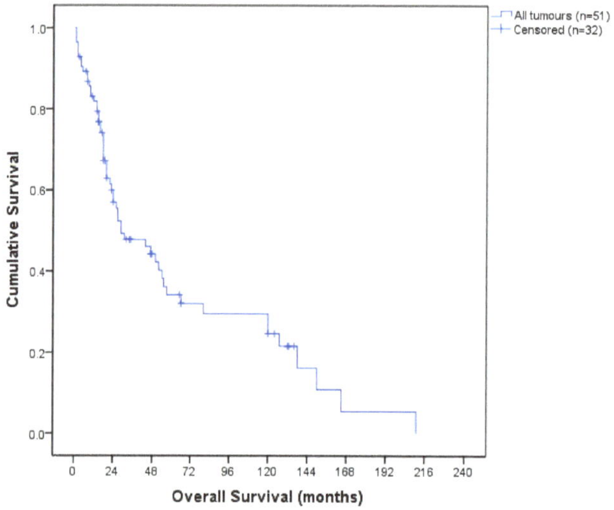

Figure 2. Overall survival curve.

3.3.1. Survival Outcomes According to Tumour Origin

We analysed survival outcomes in the two main tumours of the series, colorectal and ovarian. Curves are shown in Figures 3 and 4.

Colorectal median DFS was 19 months with a 12- and 36-month DFS of 55.7% and 39.8%, respectively; and median OS was 29 months, with a 12- and 36-month OS of 86.1% and 48.3%, respectively.

Ovarian median DFS was 15 months with a 12- and 36- month DFS of 65.5% and 31%, respectively; and median OS was 50 months, with a 12- and 36- month OS of 84.1% and 54.8%, respectively.

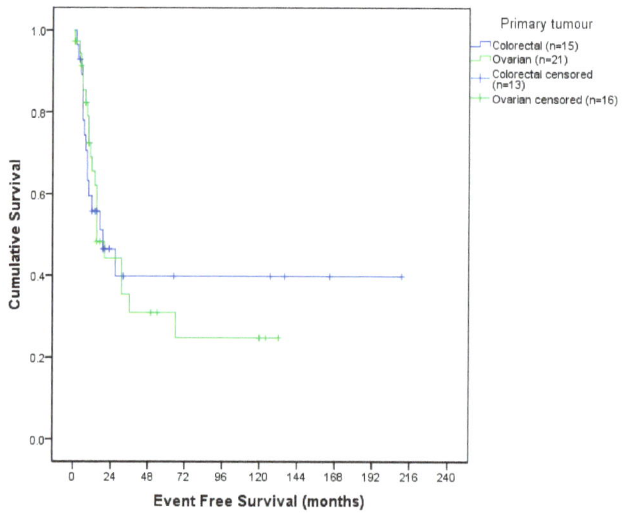

Figure 3. Ovarian and colorectal disease-free survival curve.

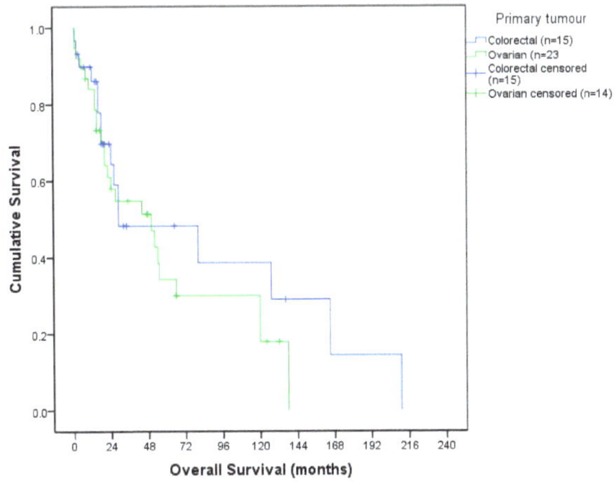

Figure 4. Ovarian and colorectal overall survival curve.

3.3.2. Survival Outcomes According to PCI

Colorectal and ovarian OS according to PCI are shown in Tables 3 and 4, respectively, and their corresponding OS curves can be seen in Figures 5 and 6.

Table 3. Colorectal overall survival according to PCI.

PCI	*n*	Median OS	12 Months OS	36 Months OS	120 Months OS
0	6	127 months	100%	55.6%	55.6%
1–9	12	80 months	91.7%	56.2%	37.5%
10–19	2	16 months	66.7%	33.3%	33.3%
≥20	6	29 months	66.7%	0%	0%

Table 4. Ovarian overall survival according to PCI.

PCI	*n*	Median OS	12 Months OS	36 Months OS	120 Months OS
0	10	20 months	90%	48%	16%
1–9	13	50 months	85.1%	61.9%	24.8%
10–19	8	44 months	87.5%	54.7%	18.2%
≥20	5	22 months	60%	30%	30%

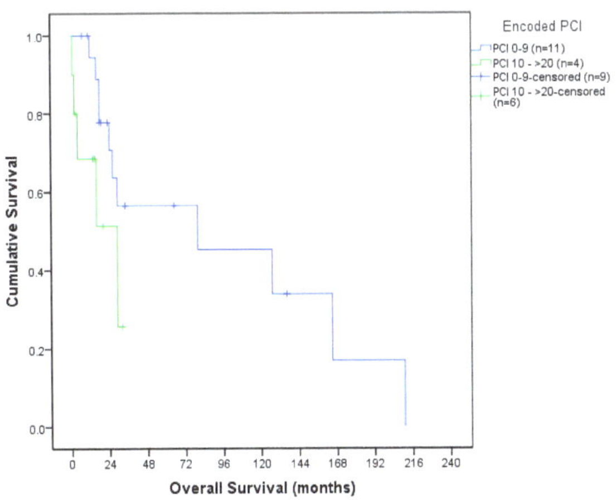

Figure 5. Colorectal overall survival curve according to PCI.

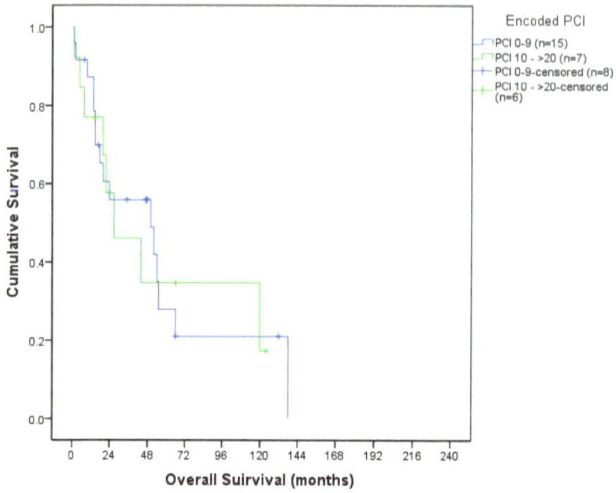

Figure 6. Ovarian overall survival curve according to PCI.

When analysing the OS curves, we combined PCI 0 with PCI 1–9 and PCI 10–19 with PCI $\geq$ 20 to obtain more statistical power, since no differences were found in survival when comparing the four groups separately. Still, we did not reach statistical significance.

3.3.3. Survival Outcomes According to CCS

Colorectal OS according to CCS is shown in Table 5 and its corresponding OS curve in Figure 7, while ovarian OS according to CCS is shown in Table 6 and its corresponding OS curve in Figure 8.

Table 5. Colorectal overall survival according to CCS.

CCS	*n*	Median OS	12 Months OS	36 Months OS	120 Months OS
CC-0	21	80 months	94.7%	59.2%	47.5%
CC-1	4	29 months	75%	0%	0%
CC-2	5	16 months	60%	30%	30%
CC-3	0	-	-	-	-

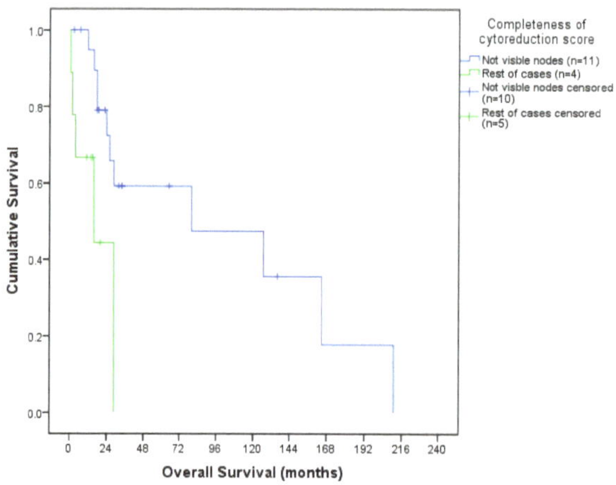

Figure 7. Colorectal overall survival curve according to CCS.

Table 6. Ovarian overall survival according to CCS.

CCS	*n*	Median OS	12 Months OS	36 Months OS	120 Months OS
CC-0	32	50 months	84.7%	51.3%	23.1%
CC-1	3	44 months	100%	100%	0%
CC-2	1	8 months *	0% *	0% *	0% *
CC-3	1	120 months *	100% *	100% *	0% *

* Data with one case only.

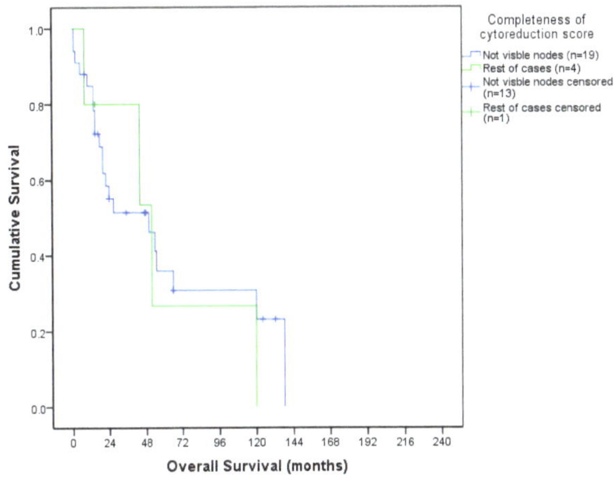

Figure 8. Ovarian overall survival curve according to CCS.

When calculating the curves, we combined CCS 0 with CCS 1 and CCS2 with CCS3 to obtain more statistical power. In colorectal patients, the comparison of the two survival curves by Log Rank Test showed a statistically significant difference ($X^2 = 4.411$; $p = 0.036$): patients with no visible nods (CCS 0 and CCS 1) had better OS curve than patients with visible nodes (CCS 2 and CCS 3). In ovarian patients, no statistical differences were found between groups.

4. Discussion

To our knowledge, this is the first study to be published in which long-term survival in patients with PM undergoing CRS +/− HIPEC is evaluated and all patients included (100%) have 10 or more years of follow-up. We obtained a global overall survival (OS) rate of 33.7% and an ovarian OS of 30%. These results are superior to the results published by Kyang et al. [12] who published an OS rate of 8%, and Kim et al. [14] who published an ovarian OS of 19.3%; but similar to the OS rate published by Ntatsis et al. [13], which was 39%. However, in these studies, the follow-up periods are heterogeneous, and some patients included do not have a 10-year follow-up period. Specifically, in Kim et al. [14] study, 14.7% of patients had less than 10 years of follow up and Kyang et al. [12] and Ntatsis et al. [13] included patients that underwent surgery until 2018 and 2019, respectively.

When analysing our survival results, it is important to remark that patients included in our study had a PCI that ranged from 0 to 39. In the early 2000s, we knew that the successful management of peritoneal metastases relied on several factors such as the presence of comorbidities, the disease stage, the tumour biology or the completeness of cancer excision [18]. In 2004, Glehen et al. [4] identified the limited extent of PCI as a positive prognostic independent factor. Ten years later, in 2014, Cascales et al. [19] published an article in which factors associated with a poor perioperative outcome were analysed and a PCI upper than 12 (OR = 2.942 95%: 1.892–9.594 $p = 0.044$) was an independent factor associated with postoperative morbidity. More recently, in 2022, van Stein et al. [20] concluded that the extent of peritoneal metastases is an independent predictor for completeness of CRS and has independent prognostic value for progression-free survival and overall survival. This evidence is consistent with our results, since we obtained lower OS rates in patients with higher PCI and higher CCS, both in colorectal and ovarian patients, even though, we only reach significance in colorectal patients when comparing CCS, probably due to our small sample. But this proves the impact of tumour burden, represented by PCI, and an adequate cytoreductive surgery, represented by CCS. Moreover, our complete cytoreduction rate (CC-0) of 80% can also explain our OS rate despite our wide PCI range, since incomplete cytoreduction has a negative influence on survival [20,21].

As far as PCI 0 patients are concerned, we should point out that the vast majority were ovarian patients treated with neoadjuvant chemotherapy in which CRS + HIPEC was a consolidation treatment being the last session of chemotherapy; or were high-risk colorectal patients in which a second-look surgery was scheduled to diagnose PM before having analytical or radiological evidence of recurrent disease. Patients with a colorectal tumour with synchronous and localized PM removed, with resected ovarian metastases or with a perforated tumour during first surgery, were considered high risk. In those patients, following the data available at that moment from prospective non-randomized studies, HIPEC with Oxaliplatin for 30 min was administered after a complete exploration of the abdominal cavity. Now, after the Prophylochip trial's publication in 2020 [22], we know that systematic second-look surgery plus oxaliplatin does not improve DFS compared to standard surveillance, and, as a consequence, now we do not perform second-look surgery in these patients as a standard of care. The rest of the PCI 0 patients were four locally advanced gastric tumours with positive cytology during the first surgery in which a second-look surgery was scheduled after neoadjuvant chemotherapy, and one mesothelioma, which was referred from another center to perform a second-look surgery.

Even though our experience in CRS and HIPEC has evolved and improved over the last two decades, the major morbidity rate (27.9%) and mortality rate (2.3%) obtained, were already consistent with the morbimortality rates published thereafter [23,24], and that was similar to other major abdominal oncological surgeries such as Whipple's procedure, esophagectomy or hepatectomy [25]. Another point to be considered when discussing morbimortality is the fact that patients included until 2008 underwent early postoperative intraperitoneal chemotherapy (EPIC) after CRS + HIPEC. This procedure required that patients remained in the intensive care unit on postoperative days 1 to 5, receiving chemotherapy through abdominal drains [26]. This technique enabled to deliver chemotherapy at the peritoneal surface to eliminate any residual microscopic tumour cells before the formation of adhesions. Unfortunately, postoperative complications such as fistula were more frequent, and long-term OS was worse than in patients receiving only HIPEC [6,27]. Consequently, EPIC could have impacted negatively in our survival rate and morbidity results, since 83.7% of our patients received EPIC. In fact, we published our results at that time and we obtained a 5-year OS of 30% with a morbidity of 40% [28].

The main limitation of our study lies in its retrospective nature, although no prospective long-term studies have been published addressing OS in PM. Another limitation is the small sample used (less than 100 patients) which was gathered from a single center and includes different origins of peritoneal metastases. Our main strength is the long-term follow-up as well as its consistency since all patients included had 10 or more years of follow-up.

To sum up, considering the historical context in which our specialized unit was founded, where patients with PM only received palliative care and CRS + HIPEC was being implemented around the world by a few centers, we conclude that CRS + HIPEC was a valid option. We obtained a morbimortality rate comparable to other major abdominal surgeries and promising survival rates, since, after 10 years of real follow-up, almost one-third of our patients are still alive and disease-free.

Author Contributions: Conceptualization, P.B.-B. and J.F.-A.; methodology, P.B.-B. and A.F.-C.; formal analysis, J.C.R.R.; investigation, P.B.-B., A.P., P.M. and A.F.-C.; data curation, A.P., P.M. and A.F.-C.; founding—M.A.O. and M.Á.-M.; writing—original draft preparation, P.B.-B., A.F.-C. and J.C.R.R.;

writing—review and editing, P.B.-B. and A.F.-C. All authors have read and agreed to the published version of the manuscript.

Funding: This research received no external funding.

Institutional Review Board Statement: The study was conducted in accordance with the Declaration of Helsinki, and approved by the Institutional Review Board of Hospital Quironsalud Torrevieja (protocol code REG-COP-2020-01 and date of approval 19 January 2021)."

Informed Consent Statement: Informed consent was obtained from all subjects involved in the study.

Data Availability Statement: The data presented in this study are available on request from the corresponding author. The data are not publicly available due to privacy restrictions.

Acknowledgments: This research was coordinated by ProA Capital, Halekulani S.L., MJR. co-financed by the European Development Regional Fund 'A way to achieve Europe', as well as P2022/BMD-7321 (Comunidad de Madrid).

Conflicts of Interest: The authors declare no conflict of interest.

References

1. Chu, D.Z.J.; Lang, N.P.; Thompson, C.; Osteen, P.K.; Westbrook, K.C. *Peritoneal carcinomatosis* in nongynecological malignancy: A prospective study of prognostic factors. *Cancer* **1989**, *63*, 364–367. [CrossRef] [PubMed]
2. Kober, F.; Heiss, A.; Roka, R. Diffuse and gross peritoneal carcinomatosis treated by intraperitoneal hyperthermic chemoperfusion. In *Peritoneal Carcinomatosis: Principles of Management*; Sugarbaker, P.H., Ed.; Kluwer Academic Publishers: Boston, MA, USA, 1996; pp. 211–219.
3. Sadeghi, B.; Arvieux, C.; Glehen, O.; Beaujard, A.C.; Rivoire, M.; Baulieux, J.; Fontaumard, E.; Brachet, A.; Caillot, J.L.; Faure, J.L.; et al. *Peritoneal carcinomatosis* from nongynecological malignancies: Results of the EVOCAPE 1 multicentric prospective study. *Cancer* **2000**, *88*, 358–363. [CrossRef]
4. Jayne, D.G.; Fook, S.; Loi, C.; Seow-Choen, F. Peritoneal carcinomatosis from colorectal cancer. *Br. J. Surg.* **2002**, *89*, 1545–1550. [CrossRef] [PubMed]
5. Verwaal, V.J.; van Ruth, S.; de Bree, E.; van Sloothen, G.W.; van Tinteren, H.; Boot, H.; Zoetmulder, F.A. Randomized trial of cytoreduction and hyperthermic intraperitoneal chemotherapy versus systemic chemotherapy and palliative surgery in patients with peritoneal carcinomatosis of colorectal cancer. *J. Clin. Oncol.* **2003**, *21*, 3737–3743. [CrossRef] [PubMed]
6. Glehen, O.; Kwiatkowski, F.; Sugarbaker, P.H.; Elias, D.; Levine, E.A.; De Simone, M.; Barone, R.; Yonemura, Y.; Cavaliere, F.; Quenet, F.; et al. Cytoreductive surgery combined with perioperative intraperitoneal chemotherapy for the management of peritoneal carcinomatosis from colorectal cancer: A multi-institutional study. *J. Clin. Oncol.* **2004**, *22*, 3284–3292. [CrossRef] [PubMed]
7. Raspagliesi, F.; Kusamura, S.; Campos Torres, J.C.; de Souza, G.A.; Ditto, A.; Zanaboni, F.; Younan, R.; Baratti, D.; Mariani, L.; Laterza, B.; et al. Cytoreduction combined with intraperitoneal hyperthermic perfusion chemotherapy in advanced/recurrent ovarian cancer patients: The experience of National Cancer Institute of Milan. *Eur. J. Surg. Oncol.* **2006**, *32*, 671–675. [CrossRef] [PubMed]
8. Glehen, O.; Schreiber, V.; Cotte, E.; Sayag-Beaujard, A.C.; Osinsky, D.; Freyer, G.; François, Y.; Vignal, J.; Gilly, F.N. Cytoreductive surgery and intraperitoneal chemohyperthermia for peritoneal carcinomatosis arising from gastric cancer. *Arch. Surg.* **2004**, *139*, 20–26. [CrossRef]
9. Marchettini, P.; Sugarbaker, P.H. Mucinous adenocarcinoma of the small bowel with peritoneal seeding. *Eur. J. Surg. Oncol.* **2002**, *28*, 19–23. [CrossRef]
10. Sugarbaker, P.H. Cytoreduction including total gastrectomy for pseudomyxoma peritonei. *Br. J. Surg.* **2002**, *89*, 208–212. [CrossRef]
11. Gómez Portilla, A.; Barrios, P.; Rufian, S.; Camps, B.; Bretcha, P.; Gonzalez Bayon, L.; Torres Melero, J.; García Polavieja, M.; Gonzalez Moreno, S. Management of peritoneal surface malignancy with cytoreductive surgery and perioperative intraperitoneal chemotherapy. *Eur. J. Surg. Oncol.* **2006**, *32*, 628–631. [CrossRef]
12. Kyang, L.S.; Alzahrani, N.A.; Valle, S.J.; Rahman, M.K.; Arrowaili, A.; Liauw, W.; Morris, D.L. Long-term survival outcomes of cytoreductive surgery and perioperative intraperitoneal chemotherapy: Single-institutional experience with 1225 cases. *J. Surg. Oncol.* **2019**, *120*, 794–802. [CrossRef] [PubMed]
13. Ntatsis, K.; Papantoni, E.; Kyziridis, D.; Kalakonas, A.; Hristakis, C.; Tzavara, C.; Tentes, A.A. Ovarian cancer: 20-year experience with cytoreductive surgery and perioperative intraperitoneal chemotherapy. *J. BUON* **2021**, *26*, 1754–1761. [PubMed]
14. Kim, S.R.; Kotsopoulos, J.; Sun, P.; Bernardini, M.Q.; Laframboise, S.; Ferguson, S.E.; Rosen, B.; Narod, S.A.; May, T. The impacts of neoadjuvant chemotherapy and of cytoreductive surgery on 10-year survival from advanced ovarian cancer. *Int. J. Gynaecol. Obstet.* **2021**, *153*, 417–423. [CrossRef] [PubMed]
15. Dindo, D.; Demartines, N.; Clavien, P.A. Classification of surgical complications: A new proposal with evaluation in a cohort of 6336 patients and results of a survey. *Ann. Surg.* **2004**, *240*, 205–213. [CrossRef] [PubMed]

16. Jacquet, P.; Sugarbaker, P.H. Current methodologies for clinical assessment of patients with peritoneal carcinomatosis. *J. Exp. Clin. Cancer Res.* **1996**, *15*, 49–58.
17. Elias, D.; Pocard, M.; Goere, D. HIPEC with oxaliplatin in the treatment of peritoneal carcinomatosis of colorectal origin. *Cancer Treat. Res.* **2007**, *134*, 303–318. [CrossRef] [PubMed]
18. Carmigani, C.P.; Esquivel, J.; Sugarbaker, P.H. Cytoreductive surgery and intraperitoneal chemotherapy for the treatment of peritoneal surface malignancy. *Rev. Oncol.* **2003**, *5*, 192–198. [CrossRef]
19. Cascales Campos, P.; Gil, J.; Parrilla, P. Morbidity and mortality outcomes of cytoreductive surgery and hyperthermic intraperitoneal chemotherapy in patients with primary and recurrent advanced ovarian cancer. *Eur. J. Surg. Oncol.* **2014**, *40*, 970–975. [CrossRef]
20. van Stein, R.M.; Engbersen, M.P.; Stolk, T.; Lopez-Yurda, M.; Lahaye, M.J.; Beets-Tan, R.G.H.; Lok, C.A.R.; Sonke, G.S.; Van Driel, W.J. Peroperative extent of peritoneal metastases affects the surgical outcome and survival in advanced ovarian cancer. *Gynecol. Oncol.* **2022**, *167*, 269–276. [CrossRef]
21. Narasimhan, V.; Tan, S.; Kong, J.; Pham, T.; Michael, M.; Ramsay, R.; Warrier, S.; Heriot, A. Prognostic factors influencing survival in patients undergoing cytoreductive surgery with hyperthermic intraperitoneal chemotherapy for isolated colorectal peritoneal metastases: A systematic review and meta-analysis. *Colorectal Dis.* **2020**, *22*, 1482–1495. [CrossRef]
22. Goéré, D.; Glehen, O.; Quenet, F.; Guilloit, J.M.; Bereder, J.M.; Lorimier, G.; Thibaudeau, E.; Ghouti, L.; Pinto, A.; Tuech, J.J.; et al. Second-look surgery plus hyperthermic intraperitoneal chemotherapy versus surveillance in patients at high risk of developing colorectal peritoneal metastases (PROPHYLOCHIP-PRODIGE 15): A randomised, phase 3 study. *Lancet Oncol.* **2020**, *21*, 1147–1154. [CrossRef] [PubMed]
23. Elias, D.; Goéré, D.; Dumont, F.; Honoré, C.; Dartigues, P.; Stoclin, A.; Malka, D.; Boige, V.; Ducreux, M. Role of hyperthermic intraoperative peritoneal chemotherapy in the management of peritoneal metastases. *Eur. J. Cancer* **2014**, *50*, 332–340. [CrossRef] [PubMed]
24. Chua, T.C.; Saxena, A.; Schellekens, J.F.; Liauw, W.; Yan, T.D.; Fransi, S.; Zhao, J.; Morris, D.L. Morbidity and mortality outcomes of cytoreductive surgery and perioperative intraperitoneal chemotherapy at a single tertiary institution: Towards a new perspective of this treatment. *Ann. Surg.* **2010**, *251*, 101–106. [CrossRef] [PubMed]
25. Foster, J.M.; Sleightholm, R.; Patel, A.; Shostrom, V.; Hall, B.; Neilsen, B.; Bartlett, D.; Smith, L. Morbidity and mortality rates following cytoreductive surgery combined with hyperthermic intraperitoneal chemotherapy compared with other high-risk surgical oncology procedures. *JAMA Netw. Open* **2019**, *2*, e186847. [CrossRef] [PubMed]
26. Sugarbaker, P.H.; Graves, T.; DeBruijn, E.A.; Cunliffe, W.J.; Mullins, R.E.; Hull, W.E.; Oliff, L.; Schlag, P. Early postoperative intraperitoneal chemotherapy as an adjuvant therapy to surgery for peritoneal carcinomatosis from gastrointestinal cancer: Pharmacological studies. *Cancer Res.* **1990**, *50*, 5790–5794. [PubMed]
27. Elias, D.; Benizri, E.; Di Pietrantonio, D.; Menegon, P.; Malka, D.; Raynard, B. Comparison of two kinds of intraperitoneal chemotherapy following complete cytoreductive surgery of colorectal peritoneal carcinomatosis. *Ann. Surg. Oncol.* **2007**, *14*, 509–514. [CrossRef] [PubMed]
28. Bretcha-Boix, P.; Farré-Alegre, J.; Sureda, M.; Dussan, C.; Pérez Ruixo, J.J.; Brugarolas Masllorens, A. Cytoreductive surgery and perioperative intraperitoneal chemotherapy in patients with peritoneal carcinomatosis of colonic origin: Outcomes after 7 years' experience of a new center for peritoneal surface malignancies. *Clin. Transl. Oncol.* **2010**, *12*, 437–442. [CrossRef]

MDPI AG
Grosspeteranlage 5
4052 Basel
Switzerland
Tel.: +41 61 683 77 34

Journal of Clinical Medicine Editorial Office
E-mail: jcm@mdpi.com
www.mdpi.com/journal/jcm

www.ingramcontent.com/pod-product-compliance
Lightning Source LLC
Chambersburg PA
CBHW041341210926
51850CB00013B/2949
* 9 7 8 3 7 2 5 8 4 6 0 3 0 *